Lifestyle Prescriptions®

Organ-Mind-Brain Yoga

There's a yoga pose for every
organ in your body

Johannes R. Fisslinger

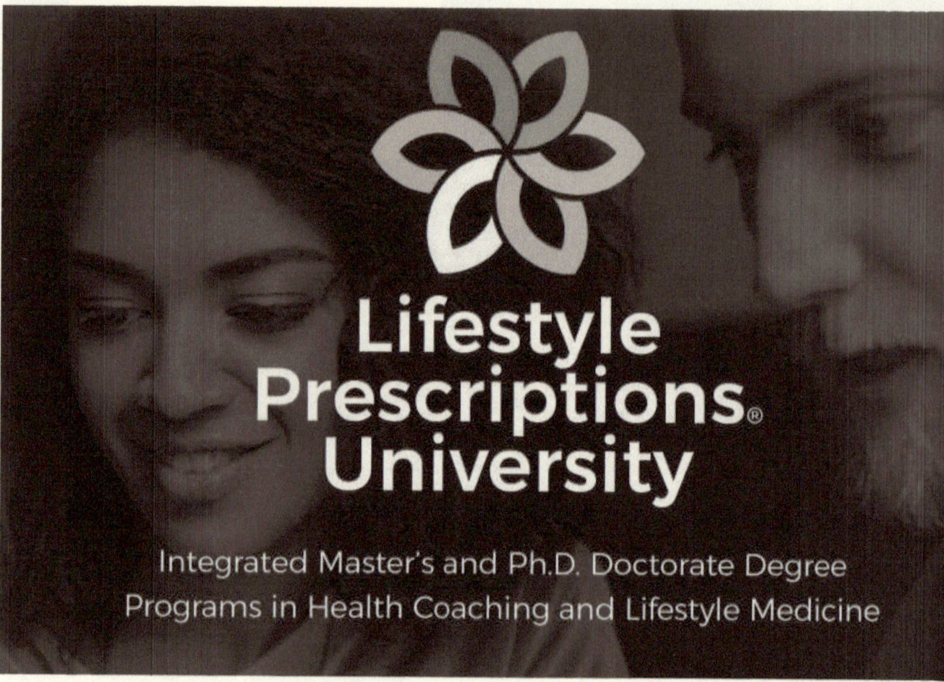

The Lifestyle Prescriptions University is the world's only Lifestyle Prescriptions® Training School and the first university exclusively focused on certificate and degree programs in root-cause based Health Coaching and Lifestyle Medicine through its innovative and high quality global long-distance programs.

Earn the following degrees and credentials:

- Ph.D. Doctorate Degree in Health Coaching and Lifestyle Medicine

- Integrated Master's Degree in Health Coaching

- Lifestyle Prescriptions® Health Coach Certificate Training

Explore how you can apply your existing health professional or yoga credentials, previous study credits and life experience to earn a degree in Root-Cause Health Coaching and Lifestyle Medicine.

Request a Degree Evaluation Review

https://lifestyleprescriptions.tv/apply

How To Use This Book

This book has been written to help you use yoga poses to strengthen and vitalize specific organs as part of your personal healthy lifestyle and yoga practice.

If you are a **health professional and want to integrate Lifestyle Prescriptions® Yoga** into your teachings and work with students then we suggest to review the following complementary course and book first:

- Book "The 6 Root-Causes Of All Symptoms"
  Download at https://lifestyleprescriptions.tv/book

- Lifestyle Prescriptions® 101 Video Course
  Watch at: https://lifestyleprescriptions.tv/101

Both are essential pre-requisites to integrate:

- The Art and Science of Self-Healing

- Organ-Mind-Brain Anatomy

- How every organ tissue in our body is linked to a specific stress trigger, emotion, belief & lifestyle habits.

- Write root-cause based Lifestyle Prescriptions® for clients and yoga students.

Organ-Mind-Brain Anatomy

The foundation of Lifestyle Prescriptions® Organ-Mind-Brain Yoga is the understanding that every organ tissue in your body is connected to a specific biological conflict, stressor, emotion, belief & lifestyle habit and a specific brain relay.

Every organ tissue in your body:

- has a biological purpose and function with the aim to help you deal with "life" (e.g. the small intestine relates to processing "food-emotions-beliefs-chunks" or the skin-epidermis is supporting you with "Loss-of-touch/Separation-Conflicts").

- displays different symptoms in stress and regeneration as part of the natural self-healing process

- will radically improve function if we give it conscious attention while staying present and mindful.

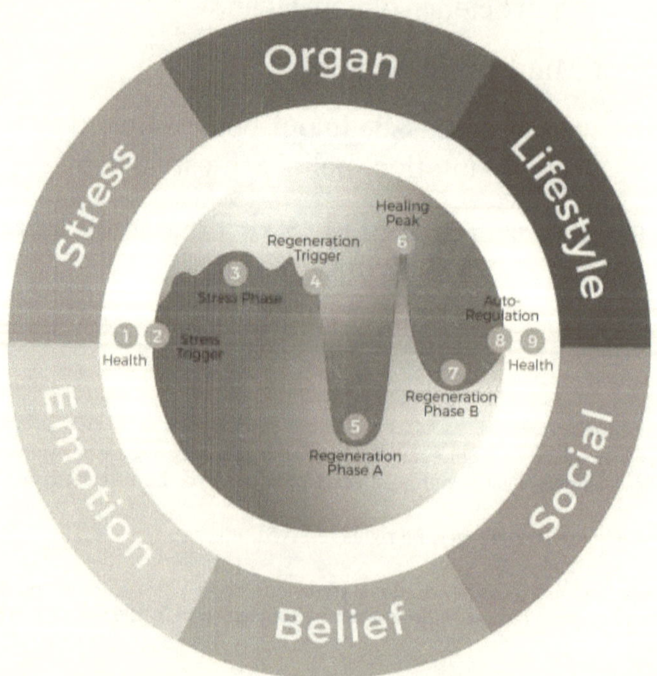

Visit www.facebook.com/lifestyleprescriptionsyoga or www.lifestyleprescriptions.tv/yoga for free videos and classes.

How To Use Yoga Poses

1. Choose a yoga pose and practice that pose for 7 days daily (you can choose a stand-alone practice or integrate that pose into your existing yoga practice).

2. For example, if you or a client has digestive symptoms then practicing a yoga pose that strengthens and vitalizes the digestive track.

3. After 7 days continue, select a new or add another pose.

4. While practicing a yoga pose be present; feel "breath-prana-life force" flow into the organ tissue you're about to awaken.

5. At the same time let go of any emotion or thought that might appear. With every exhale feel unresolved emotional hurts and limiting beliefs flow out of that organ tissue.

6. Return your attention again and again into the organ tissue. With every inhale feel, see, hear light, love and pure consciousness expand and with every exhale release old and unwanted energies.

7. Most important enjoy!

Table Of Content

Yoga Poses By Anatomy

Poses For Arms

Crow Pose

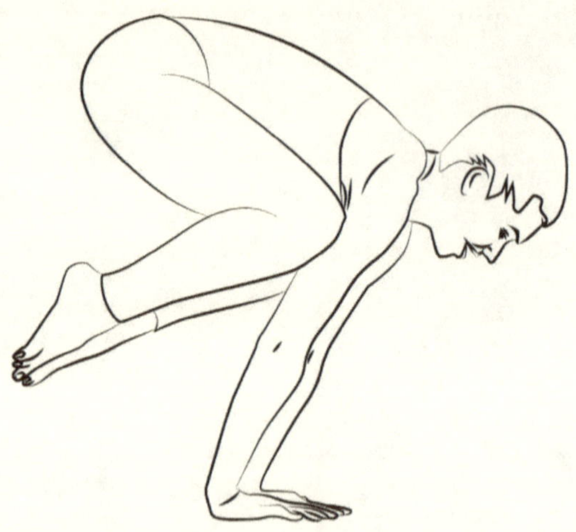

The crow pose is an arm balancing asana and a bit more advanced, but beginners can practice the easier variation, which will, with some practice, allow you to master it. This pose looks harder than it is, so don't be intimidated. It's more about coordination and concentration and not so much about your upper body strength.

Organs:

- ➢ Arms
- ➢ Shoulders
- ➢ Wrists
- ➢ Organs in the abdomen

Benefits:

The crow pose tones your arms and the abdominal wall, relieving lower back pain and strengthening the digestive organs.

This asana also stretches and tones your back muscles and inner thighs and opens the groin.

Beginner tips:

Attempt this pose slowly, giving yourself plenty of time. At first just stick to rocking back and forth, lifting just one foot at a time, developing your balance and strengthening the muscles in your wrists, arms and shoulders. After some time and practice you can attempt to take the other foot off the ground and try balancing yourself on your arms, even if only for a second, and gradually build on the pose from there.

Steps:

To make this pose easier to get into, place a yoga block on your mat and step onto it.

Bend your knees and separate them into a comfortable squat and plant your palms firmly on your mat with your fingers spread wide.

Push your knees towards the outer edges of your arms and squeeze them around the arms.

Try not to look straight down but keep your gaze a little bit in front of you. Lift your heels and place the weight onto the balls of your feet. Keep your elbows directly over the wrists.

Rock back and forth, shifting your weight onto the hands to get warmed up. When you feel confident enough, raise one toe off the floor and then the other, pressing against your hands.

Touch your toes behind you. Round your upper body and attempt to straighten the arms as if you're pushing the ground away.

Take a deep breath and gently lower yourself back into the squat position.

Therapeutic Applications:

It helps you build endurance and focus; you are balancing your entire body on your hands and that's no piece of cake!

Improves your balance and concentration.

Precautions:

Do not attempt this asana if you have carpal tunnel syndrome, because this pose puts a lot of strain on your wrists.

Also avoid this pose if you are pregnant or are suffering from high blood pressure.

Downward Facing Dog Pose

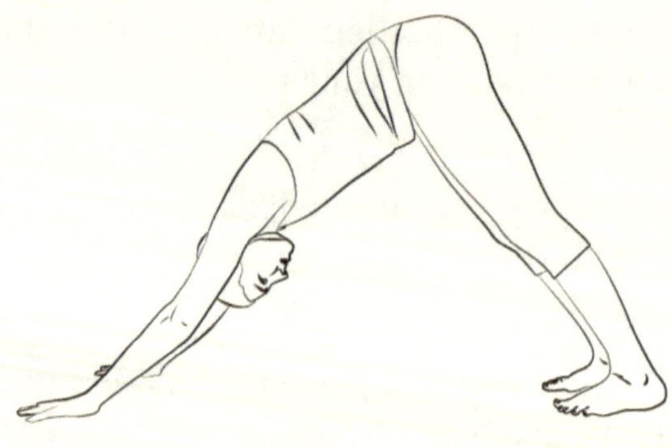

The Downward facing dog is one of the most widely recognized poses in yoga and gets its name from the way dogs tend to stretch their bodies. It's a great pose for decompressing the spine and creating a feeling of openness in your body. It is also one of the key poses in the Sun Salutation yoga routine. This asana stretches and energizes your entire body while calming your mind and toning your arms and legs.

Organs:

> Arm muscles

> Leg muscles

> Abdomen

Benefits:

The downward facing dog has numerous beneficial effects for your mind and body. It calms the brain and helps you battle stress and mild forms of depression.

It energizes the body and prevents headaches, insomnia and fatigue.

The pose strengthens the shoulders, hamstrings, calves and hands and tones your arms and legs.

Beginner tips:

Beginners might find it difficult to open up their shoulders. In this case try lifting your hands off the floor on a pair of yoga blocks.

Don't feel bad if your heels don't touch the floor, as long as they're reaching downward it's perfectly fine. Avoid walking your feet closer to your hands to achieve this effect.

Steps:

Begin lying on your stomach on your mat and place your fingertips in line with the centre of your chest.

Push yourself up, keeping your wrists under your shoulders and your knees below your hips.

Then tuck your toes and raise your hips toward the ceiling so that your body forms the inverted letter "V".

The most crucial part in the downward facing dog pose is to find the appropriate distance between your hands and feet. Straighten your knees and lift your hips even higher and press your heels towards the floor.

The fronts of your wrists should be parallel to the mat, your fingers spread and pressing into the mat as if digging into sand.

Extend your arms and straighten your elbows. Press your shoulder blades towards your back and widen them.

The downward facing dog is the perfect position for steadying your breath. Take your time and stay in this pose for a few deep breaths. To release, simply lower your knees to the floor and into the relaxing child's pose.

Therapeutic Applications:

Doing this pose regularly has therapeutic effects for those with high blood pressure, asthma, flat feet and sciatica.

Precautions:

If you're suffering from carpal tunnel syndrome or have diarrhoea, you should avoid this asana.

Pregnant women should also avoid doing the downwards facing dog in the third trimester.

If you have high blood pressure or are suffering from a headache, just support your head on a block and keep your ears level between the arms.

Plank And Side-Plank Pose

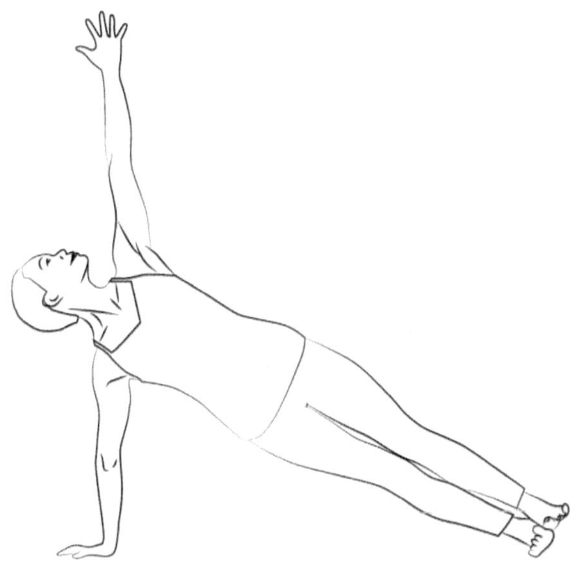

The plank pose is a simple beginner-friendly pose and one of the essential asanas in the traditional Sun Salutation yoga routine. It is said that sometimes the simplest of exercises have the greatest benefits and the plank pose is no exception. It is one of the best poses to improve core strength while allowing you to maintain a straight and stable spine, toning your arms in the process.

Organs:

- ➢ Arms

- ➢ Abdomen

- ➢ Back muscles

- ➢ Strenthens the core muscles

Benefits:

The plank pose is a great way to tone the abdominal and back muscles and strengthen your core. It also works your shoulders and your arms.

Beginner tips:

Practice this pose in front of a mirror. It is important to keep your spine straight and to avoid slumping or arching your back while in this pose.

Steps:

Start in the downward facing dog pose. On the inhale, roll your upper back forward and bring the full length of your body parallel to the floor with your wrists stacked below your shoulders.

Balance yourself on the tips of your toes, all the while keeping the stomach firm.

Press your shoulder blades against your back and keep your shoulders, hips and knees is one long plank-like position and keep the top of your head in line with your spine.

If this pose is not challenging enough for you, you can try lowering yourself onto your forearms. Your elbows should be below your shoulders as your arms face forward.

For the side plank, start from the plank pose, stack your hips to the right side and slightly bend your right elbow.

Slowly shift your body to the side, transferring your weight and placing the left leg on top of the right while your left arm stretches towards the sky.

Stack your shoulders on top of your wrists and keep your body in one long straight line all the way from your feet to the top of your head and from your right wrist to the fingertips of your left hand.

Slowly shift back to the neutral plank pose and repeat the side plank on the other side as well.

Therapeutic Applications:

Improves balance.

Strengthening your body core improves your overall posture.

Precautions:

Avoid this pose if you have carpal tunnel syndrome or feel pain or discomfort in your wrists.

The side-plank pose is even more strenuous on your arms, shoulders and wrist so avoid this asana if you have problems with these areas of your body.

Upward Facing Dog Pose

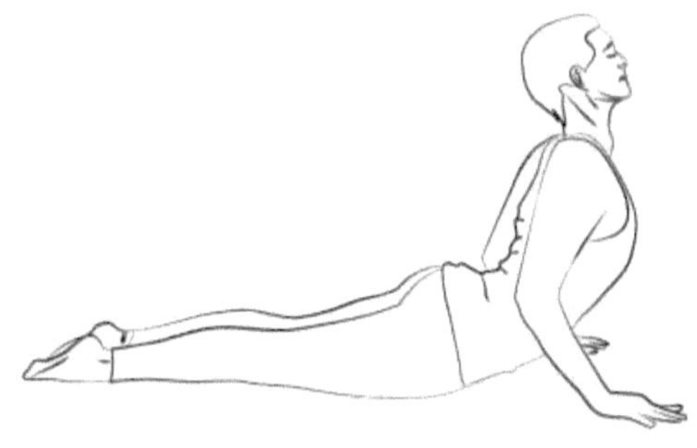

The upward facing dog is a very powerful pose that strengthens and awakens the entire upper part of your body and offers a refreshing stretch to the chest and abdomen. This pose should be done carefully, because often one misaligned body part can cause a domino effect for the entire pose, so you should really check the beginner tips on how to avoid that. But when done properly, this asana strengthens your entire body and tones your arms.

Organs:

> Arms

> Back muscles

> Abdomen

> Chest

Benefits:

When practiced correctly, the upward facing dog pose opens the chest and strengthens the entire body and tones the arms.

This pose aligns the spine.

Beginner tips:

Here are three key cues that will prevent you from misaligning your body: keep the shoulders from creeping up towards the ears; do not rest the entire weight on the wrists, but press through the hands to create the sensation of a lift; and do not let your legs and knees touch the mat.

If you are having problems with this pose, try placing yoga blocks under the palms.

Steps:

Start this pose in the downward facing dog, roll your upper back forward, straighten your body into the plank pose and lower your knees to the ground.

Bend the elbows as if hugging them into the sides and lower your chest forward and down until your upper arms are parallel to the floor.

Keep your pelvis, torso, shoulders and head in one long line.

Press your shoulders down and back and draw them away from your ears.

Next, straighten your elbows and lift your chest until your shoulders are stacked directly on top of your hands and lower your hips.

Press the tops of your feet to the floor and lift your thighs. Stay here for one to three breaths.

While holding the pose, beginners should look straight ahead while more advanced practitioners can look up, without compressing the back of the neck.

To release, bend the knees and sit on your heels in the child's pose to relax.

Therapeutic Applications:

It has a therapeutic affect on the kidneys and the nervous system.

Because this pose opens up your chest and stretches the lungs, it is beneficial for those suffering from asthma

Precautions:

Avoid this pose if you are suffering from a chronic back injury or are recovering from an injury to your hips, arms, wrists or shoulders.

Do not do this pose if you are pregnant or have recently had abdominal surgery.

Poses For Knees

Chair pose

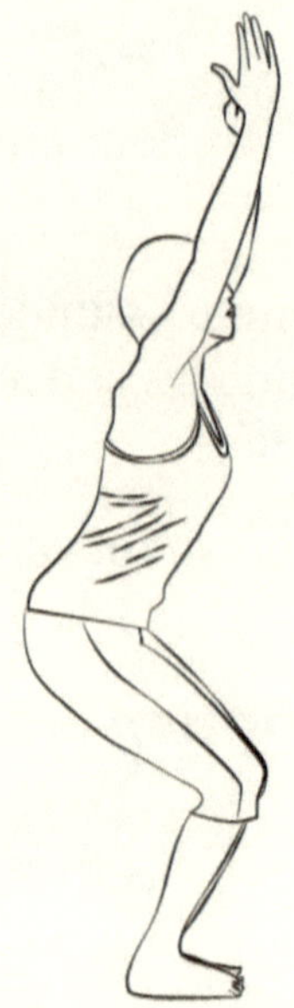

Sitting in a chair sounds like a very easy and comfortable task, but when the chair is imaginary, it might prove slightly more challenging. The chair pose is also known as the "Fierce" or "The Powerful Pose". It helps to improve strength, balance and stability while helping build endurance. This pose will not only help you gain stamina, but will strengthen the knees, hamstrings and abductor muscles and increase blood flow to the lower part of the body.

Organs:

- ➢ Knees

- ➢ Legs

- ➢ Chest

Benefits:

This asana helps prevent ankle and knee injuries.

It strengthens your thighs, calves and spine, stretches the shoulders and expands the chest.

Beginner tips:

The chair pose is typically practiced away from the wall, but if you believe your knees are not quite strong enough to support you during this pose or are feeling unsure, you can use a wall to support you during this asana.

Place your feet apart so that they are in line with your hips, lean back against the wall and slide down until your knees and hips are parallel with each other. Hold this pose for a few breaths before lifting yourself back up and repeat several times. Your arms can rest on your knees or you can stretch them out towards the sky.

If you have a yoga block, you can place it between your thighs to help the knees point forward.

Steps:

Stand in the mountain pose, and slowly start to bend your knees and lift your arms while you gently push your pelvis down as if sitting back in an imaginary chair.

Broaden the front of your chest and lift your torso.

Press your shoulders down and back, slightly arching the spine, and elongate your neck.

Gently tighten your lower abdomen and lift the front of your hip up and away from your thighs.

Try to keep your thighs as parallel to the floor as possible, but remember to never let your knees go over your feet.

Stand in this position for two to three breaths then straighten your legs back to the mountain pose and slowly lower your arms to the sides.

Therapeutic Applications:

Practicing this pose regularly stimulates abdominal organs, the heart and the diaphragm.

Precautions:

Avoid this asana if you suffer from headaches, insomnia or low blood pressure.

It is also not recommended if you have chronic knee pain, ligament problems and arthritis or are recovering from an ankle injury.

Extended side angle pose

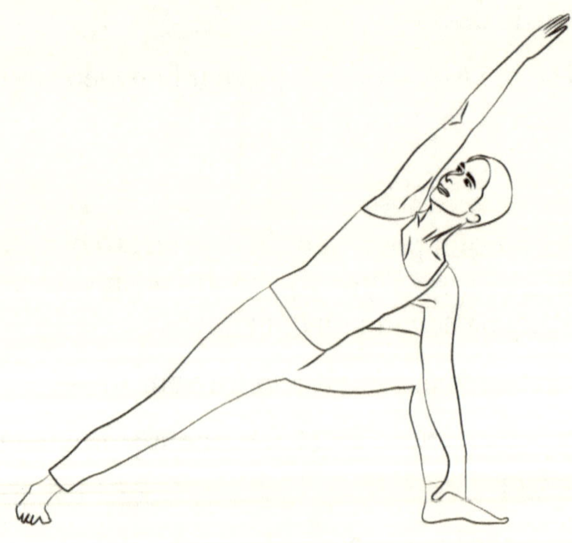

The Extended side angle pose is basically a lunge, combined a slight twisting of the spine and stretching. It's done in two parts, on the right and left side. This pose stretches the entire side of your body, which is often neglected during exercise, strengthens the legs and knees and opens the inner thighs.

Organs:

- ➢ Legs

- ➢ Knees

- ➢ Ankles

- ➢ Groin muscles

- ➢ Spine

- ➢ Chest

- ➢ Shoulders

Benefits:

It strengthens and stretches your legs, knees and ankles, it stretches the groin muscles and the spine.

It expands the chest, lungs and shoulders.

It also stimulates your abdominal muscles and increases overall stamina.

Beginner tips:

Beginners often have difficulty with keeping their back heel rooted to the floor when bending the front knee and are unable to comfortably touch the floor with the fingertips of their lower hand when in the pose. Try standing near a wall and bracing your back heel against it, as if trying to push the wall away from you.

Steps:

Begin by standing in the mountain pose and put your hands on your hips.

Step your with your feet about an arm's length apart or whatever feels comfortable.

Turn your right foot out so that it's vertical to your back (left) foot and align your heels.

Lower your hips to the ground and bend your right knee so that it is directly above your shin. Firmly root your left heel to the ground.

If you want to challenge yourself more, just place your feet further apart.

Then bend your right elbow and place your right forearm on your thigh.

Keep your spine and head aligned while gazing forward, stretching your left arm up and above your head.

Your body should form a long and straight line from the outside of your left foot to your hip, along the torso, and up the outer arm to the very fingertips of your left hand.

If this is not challenging enough for you, then place your right hand on a block behind your right foot.

After a few deep breaths, switch the position to the other side by bending the left knee and placing the left forearm on top of it.

Therapeutic Applications:

This pose relieves constipation, low backache and osteoporosis.

It helps alleviate menstrual discomfort.

Precautions:

You should avoid doing this asana if you suffer from headaches, high or low blood pressure and insomnia.

If you have any neck problems, you should avoid turning your head to face the top arm and look straight ahead or to the floor instead, with the neck elongated.

Wide-Angled Seated Forward Bend Pose

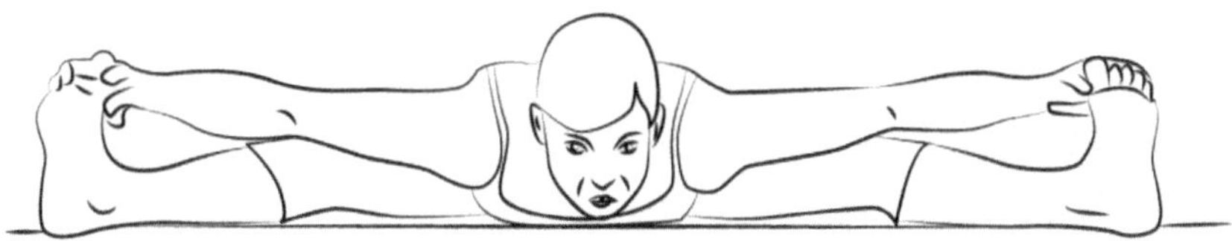

Many poses that strengthen your legs can also be stressful on the knees, which make them quite uncomfortable for those suffering from knee problems and pain. This pose is a forward bend, which means it opens the entire back of your body. This is a great pose that will stretch out your back, hips, inner thighs and groin. And because you will be sitting on the ground, you will be able to stretch the knees without putting unnecessary strain on them.

Organs:

- ➤ Thighs

- ➤ Knees

- ➤ Abdomen

- ➤ Back

- ➤ Hips

Benefits:

The wide-angled seated forward bend is great for stretching the insides and backs of the legs as well as knees.

It stimulates the abdominal organs.

It strengthens the spine.

Beginner tips:

Beginners may have trouble with this seated forward bend, so bend over as much as you can so that you still feel comfortable. But if you're having trouble bending forward even slightly, then you can bend your knees just a little to make the pose easier.

Remember to keep your knee caps always pointing to the ceiling.

If you find the forward bend too difficult, place a bolster, harder pillow or a rolled up towel straight in front of you and in line with your upper body.

Steps:

To do this pose, begin by sitting on your mat with your legs extending forward and then open your legs to the side as wide as you comfortably can, ideally it should be slightly wider than a 90-degree angle.

Keep pressing your outer thighs against the mat, while your knee caps point towards the ceiling.

Place your hands on the ground in front of you and slowly walk them forward until you can feel a comfortable stretch, all the while keeping your spine straight and elongated.

With each exhale try and increase the forward bend, so that you feel a nice stretch in the backs of your legs.

If you catch yourself bending from the waist, readjust your pose and continue forward if possible.

Therapeutic Applications:

This pose has a therapeutic affect on the kidneys.

It is very beneficial for those suffering from sciatica or arthritis.

Precautions:

If you have a lower back injury or are feeling discomfort in this region, try sitting on a folded blanket or some other prop while keeping your torso as upright as you can.

You should avoid this pose if you have pulled your hamstrings or groin muscles.

If you cannot enter and exit the pose without causing pain, then you should avoid doing it.

Half frog pose

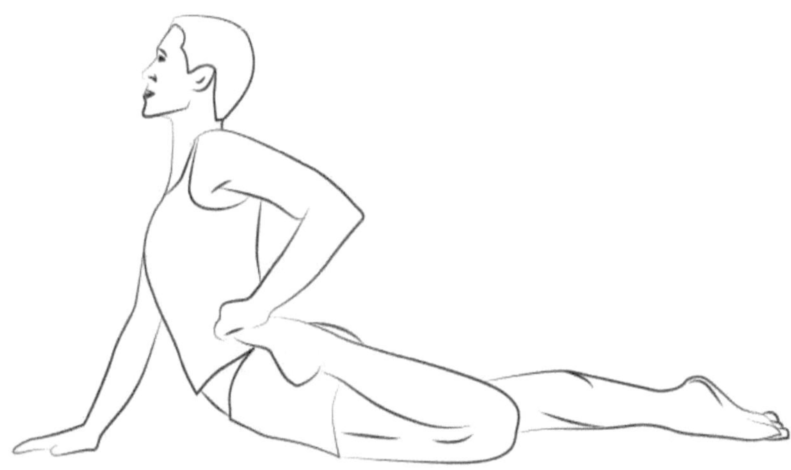

The half frog pose is an intermediate pose that is beneficial for those who can't run, dance or walk long distances because they have flat feet. It is also a highly recommended asana for runners or those engaged in outdoor sports, because it strengthens your leg muscles and reduces the chance of knee injuries when practiced regularly. The half frog pose stretches the entire front body, chest, abdomen, groin, thighs and ankles and rejuvenates the knee joints.

Organs:

- ➢ Leg muscles
- ➢ Knees
- ➢ Chest
- ➢ Abdomen
- ➢ Ankles
- ➢ Groin muscles

Benefits:

This asana stretches your ankles, thighs, groin muscles, your abdomen and the entire front of the torso.

It opens the chest and shoulders.

Doing this pose regularly strengthens your back muscles and improves your posture by reinforcing spinal column alignment.

Beginner tips:

Beginners can support the lift of the upper torso by putting a bolster under the lower ribs and pressing the free forearm on the mat in front of the bolster. If you're having problems reaching behind to catch your foot, use a strap or scarf and wrap it around your ankle.

While doing this asana, do not place all your weight on the left shoulder, but instead square your shoulders and press down with the left elbow to lift up your chest.

Steps:

To begin, lie on your yoga mat on your stomach, place your forearms on the floor and lift up your head and upper torso.

Press the pelvic bone into the mat and draw in your stomach.

Bend your right knee and pull it gently towards the side of the right buttock.

While supporting yourself on your left forearm, take your right hand and reach back to grab the inside of your foot, while still pressing your hip into the floor.

The base of your palm should press the top of the foot but be sure to keep the knee in line with your hip.

Stop immediately, if you feel any pain in your knee or elsewhere.

Try holding this pose for about a minute or at least two to three deep breaths. Release your foot and repeat the steps with the left leg.

Therapeutic Applications:

Stimulates organs in the abdomen, improving digestion.

It increases blood flow to the uterus and ovaries, giving it a therapeutic affect against infertility.

The half frog pose also relieves symptoms of menopause as well as menstrual cramps.

Precautions:

Avoid this pose if you suffer from low or high blood pressure, migraines, insomnia or have sustained any injuries to your lower back, neck or shoulders.

Child's pose

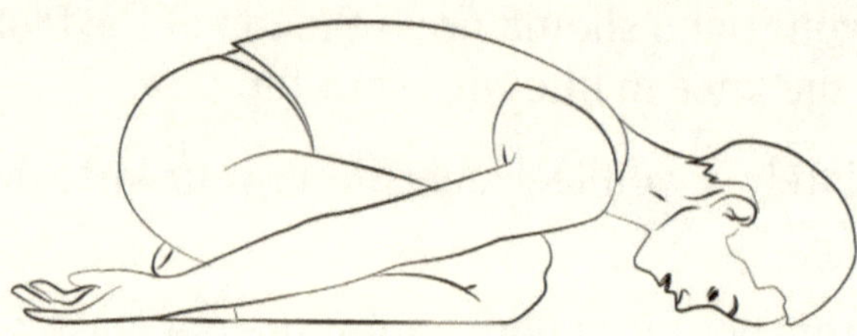

The child's pose is mainly a restorative asana, during which you relax and rest during some more difficult yoga exercises. Although it may feel like you're not doing any work, your ankles and thighs get a nice stretch.

Organs:

> Ankles

> Thighs

> Arms

Benefits:

This is a resting pose which can precede and follow any other asana. When doing a more intense yoga workout, just go to the child's pose when you're feeling tired or short of breath.

It gives your hips, ankles and thighs a nice stretch and releases tension in the back, neck, shoulders and chest.

Beginner tips:

If you're a beginner and are having a difficult time sitting on your heels, place a tightly folded blanket between the back of your thighs and calves.

Steps:

Begin this pose by kneeling on your mat with your big toes touching behind you. The tops of your feet are pressing into the mat, the toes are pointing back.

Lower yourself and sit on your heels while spreading your knees to the width of your hips. Lean forward and press your upper body into your upper thighs and rest your forehead on the mat.

Place your arms on the mat alongside your torso and let them point back with palms facing upwards. Let your shoulders simply sag to the ground.

Focus consciously on your breathing and use this asana as an opportunity to breathe into the back of your torso, imagining your spine lengthening with each inhale.

If you want to lengthen your torso and go for a more active child's pose, stretch your arms forward as if you're reaching for something, while drawing your shoulder blades back.

Therapeutic Applications:

By encouraging strong and regular breaths, the child's pose also calms the mind and helps relieve stress, anxiety, fatigue and helps to establish a normal circulation in the body.

Precautions:

You should avoid this asana if you have diarrhoea.

Pregnant women or those recovering from hip surgery can practice this pose with a slight variation: instead of bringing the knees together, keep them at least at hip distance apart.

You should also avoid this pose if you have had recent knee surgery.

Hero pose

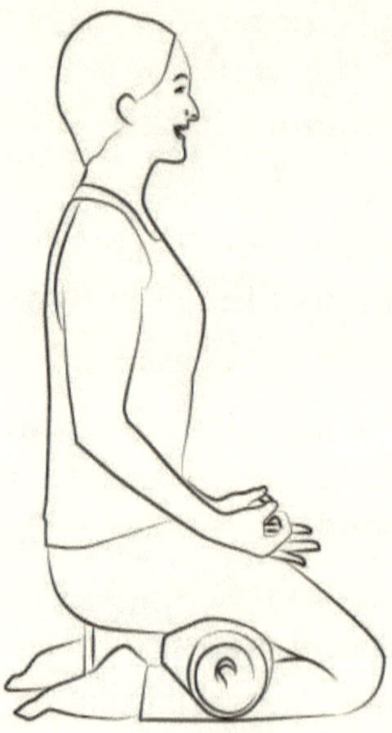

The hero pose is very similar to the lightning bolt asana and can also be an alternative pose to use for meditation. Like in the lightning pose, you sit back on your legs, only this time you slide them apart and sit between your ankles, your outer hip brushing against the inner side of your heels.

Organs:

- ➢ Legs

- ➢ Knees

- ➢ Ankles

- ➢ Back muscles

Benefits:

It keeps your knees and ankles healthy by increasing flexibility in your legs, knees, ankles and thus preventing injuries.

Strengthens and stretches your hips, thighs and feet.

Keeping a straight back also strengthens the muscles in your back and improves your overall posture.

It is also a beneficial pose for pregnant women (in the second trimester), because it helps to reduce swelling in the legs.

Beginner tips:

If this pose is too difficult and causes discomfort or pain in your upper thighs or knees, you can try using a block or a rolled-up towel and place it between your ankles. It's important that your sitting bones touch the floor, blanket or block that you are using.

Steps:

To begin this yoga pose, start by kneeling on your yoga mat, keeping your thighs horizontal to the floor.

 If you feel discomfort in your legs, place a blanket beneath your feet or knees to gently pad them.

Slide your feet apart so that they are a bit wider than the hips, but make sure your feet are in line with the shins.

Then slowly sit down between your ankles or, if you find this to challenging or feel any strain in your thighs or knees, place a block or rolled-up blanket between your feet to make it easier to sit.

The tops of your feet should stay flat and outstretched on your mat, while the inner sides of your knees should remain close together.

Keep your spine and back straight, relax your shoulders and rest your hands on your thighs.

The top of your head should point to the ceiling while looking straight ahead.

Breathe deeply and evenly for as long as it feels comfortable.

Therapeutic Applications:

Great for improving digestion.

Therapeutic for those suffering from asthma and high blood pressure.

Precautions:

Although this pose is great for strengthening the knees and ankles, you should avoid practicing the hero pose if you are suffering from a knee or ankle injury.

Lightning bolt pose

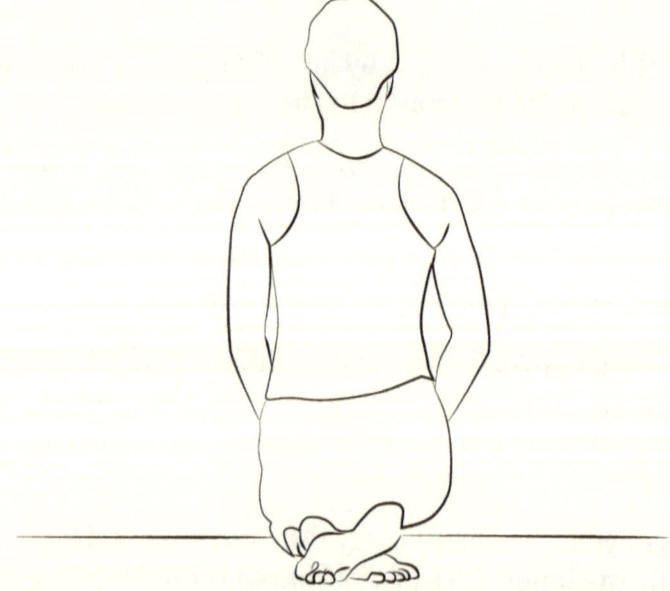

The lightning bolt pose is a very simple asana, used also as an alternative meditative pose by those, who have lower back problems and are uncomfortable sitting in the lotus pose. Simply sit back on your heels, relax and focus on your breathing and you can stay in this pose comfortably for a longer period of time.

Organs:

> Ankles

> Thighs

> Knees

> Back muscles

Benefits:

Stretching and gently massaging your ankles.

Helps strengthen muscles of the legs and back.

Beginner tips:

If your ankles feel uncomfortable during this asana, try putting a folded towel or blanket under them.

This pose is easy to do and perfect for beginners, but if you are having trouble because your legs keep sliding apart, here's a quick tip: try using a scarf or something similar to tie your ankles together (gently and not so tight it causes pain or discomfort.)

Steps:

Begin this pose by standing on your knees with your legs close together, stretching backwards.

Gently lower your body and sit down on the backs of your heels with your thighs resting on your calves. Make sure your feet don't lean out to the side and that your big toes are touching.

Keep your back straight and your head aligned with your spine, resting your hands on your thighs. Try rocking gently back and front to stretch and massage your ankles.

You can even place your palms on the floor behind you and lean back or, if you feel up to it, place the forearms and elbows on the floor behind you and lean back, arching your back slightly.

If you start to feel pain in your legs, simply stretch out your legs in front of you and gently massage them and then try again if you feel comfortable.

Therapeutic Applications:

It is a meditative pose if you feel uncomfortable in the lotus pose.

It is actually recommended to do this pose shortly after a meal. Sitting in this pose increases blood flow to the pelvic region and boosts the efficiency of the digestive tract, improving metabolism and helping with constipation.

Precautions:

You should avoid doing this asana if you have problems with your knees or are recovering from a knee surgery, because this pose puts additional stress on the knees.

Pregnant women should do this asana with their knees slightly apart in order to avoid applying too much pressure on the abdomen.

Mountain pose

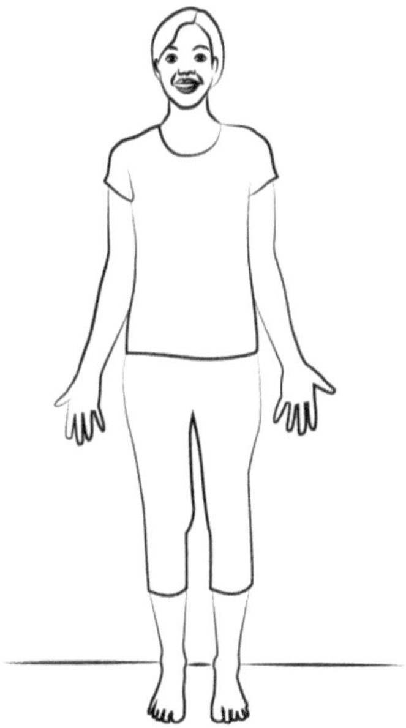

The mountain pose is a very beginner-friendly asana and a foundational pose which helps you to align and straighten your spine. Simple as it is, it has several benefits for your body. The mountain pose is often the first pose you do when starting your yoga practice, but it's also useful to practice this asana as a pose in itself. When doing it properly, you should experience a feeling as if being rooted to the ground while standing tall and motionless as a mountain.

Organs:

> Back muscles

> Abdominal muscles

> Thighs

> Knees

> Ankles

Benefits:

It trains the entire foot to support the ankle and helps you to balance your weight evenly. It also helps reverse negative side effects of poor posture.

Helps re-train the body to stand properly.

This pose also gives you a better sense of balance while strengthening your thighs, knees and ankles. It also firms your abdominal muscles as well as your buttocks.

Beginner tips:

Beginners can try to improve their balance by standing with the inner parts of the feet only slightly apart. If you want to make the pose just a little bit harder, try doing it with your eyes closed, which will really put your balance to the test.

If you are not sure whether you are aligned properly, try this pose while standing with your back against a wall. The backs of your heels and your shoulder blades should touch the wall, but not the back of your head.

Steps:

You begin by standing with your feet together, the big toes touching and heels slightly apart as you stand in a neutral position.

Release your arms alongside your body with the palms facing inward.

Elongate your spine and tailbone and align your head directly over the centre of your spine, keeping your chin parallel to the floor.

Roll back your shoulder blades and widen them, expanding your chest, while your hands hang alongside your torso. (If you want, you can stretch your arms toward the ceiling on the inhale and lowering them back on the exhale.)

Lift your sternum straight towards the sky and begin focusing on your breath and directing your attention inward.

Therapeutic Applications:

Doing this asana properly relieves sciatica.

It is beneficial for those with flat feet.

Precautions:

Because of the effects of standing, practicing this pose for a longer period of time should be done with caution or under supervision by those who suffer from headaches, insomnia or have low blood pressure.

With this asana the position of the feet is very important as even minor alterations can affect the entire posture of your body.

Bharadvaja's Twist

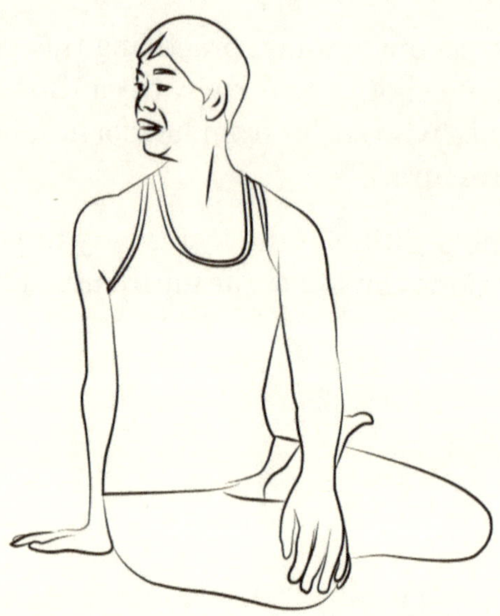

The Bharadvaja's twist is a seated yoga pose. It is a simple yoga pose which makes is ideal for beginners. It is also known as the Baharadvajasana I and regular practice of this pose has a soothing effect of the body. It also has other benefits like relaxing the nervous system and rejuvenating the spine as well as muscles of the body.

Organs

> Abdomen
> Spine
> Shoulders
> Hip

Benefits

The Bharadvaja's twist calms and restores underlying organs in the body, leading to enhanced digestive function, improved metabolic activity and superior detoxification process by promoting better elimination of waste from the body.

It calms the mind and restores a sense of balance.

It stretches the spine, shoulders and hips.

Pregnant women can also benefit from this pose because it exerts no pressure on the abdomen and strengthens the lower back especially in the second trimester.

Beginner tips

A person new to yoga could rest the buttock on a thickly folded blanket or cloth, and this would help to level out the body and ensure the weight of the body is firmly pressed against the ground.

Steps

Start by sitting on the floor with both legs stretched out in front of you, and then let your arms rest on either side.

Take both knees towards the right so that your feet drop to the left. The weight of the body should be rested firmly on the right buttock and the inner side of the left ankle should rest on the arch of the right foot.

Then place your left hand outside the right knee and the left fingertips should be on the floor behind you. Create stability by hugging in and rooting the tailbone as much as possible into the ground.

While inhaling slowly, stretch the spine to lengthen it as much as possible and then exhale while twisting the trunk to the maximum extent possible.

Next, while bending the upper back slightly, twist the spine and feel its effect along its entire length, from the tailbone to the head.

Inhale and exhale slowly, applying a lengthening force with each inhalation and twisting with each exhalation.

After this pose has been maintained for about a minute, exhale slowly while untwisting and revert back to the original position.

Repeat asana for the opposite side.

Therapeutic Applications

Massages the internal organs, improves digestion and detoxifies the body.

Relieves sciatica, lumbargo and cervicalgia.

Beneficial in carpal tunnel syndrome.

Precautions

Individuals with diarrhea and unstable blood pressure should perform this pose with caution.

Individuals with a history of spine and hip disorders should seek medical opinion before performing this pose.

Bridge Pose

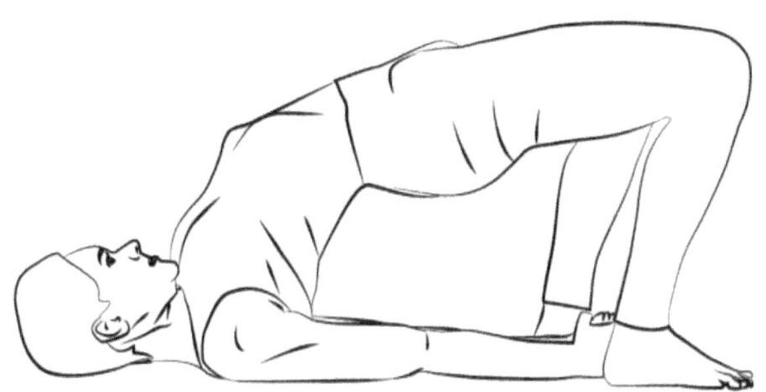

The bridge pose is also called the Setu Bandhasana. It is one of the less rigorous yoga backbend exercises and it's a gateway to the more complicated backbend poses as it improves balance and stability. The final posture this pose resembles a bridge, hence the name. It has advantageous effects on the chest, back, shoulders and lungs.

Organs

> Abdominal organs
> Lungs
> Thyroid

Benefits

It stimulates abdominal organs and helps to improve digestion.

Opens up the lungs and reduces thyroid problems.

It relieves tired back instantly.

It stretches the back muscles as well as the chest, neck and spine.

Relieves stress on the nervous system, thereby reducing stress, depression and anxiety.

Beginner's Tips

Try not to pull the shoulders forcefully away from the ears once they are rolled in, this tends to overstretch the neck. Instead, lift the tip of the shoulders towards the ears and try to push the inner part of the shoulder blades away from the spine.

You can place a thickly folded blanket beneath the shoulders to protect the neck.

Steps

Start by lying flat on the back in a supine position with both palms facing downwards.

Fold the legs at the knees and bring the feet closer to the buttock region. Ideally, your hands should be able to touch your heels.

Press your hands and shoulders firmly into the floor and you should feel the chest begin to lift. At the same time, ground the plantar surface of the feet firmly into ground.

Then slowly, while inhaling, begin to lift your buttocks away from the ground, keeping the knees directly over the heels and away from the hips to lengthen the spine. As you do this, raise the coccyx slowly and continue lifting the spine. Ideally, the tailbone should reach the level of the knees.

Next, move the chin a little away from the chest, then try to lift the chest towards the chin using the shoulder. The weight your body should now be resting on your arms, shoulders and feet.

Stay in this pose for as long as possible while breathing slowly and deeply. Ideally, it should be retained for at least a minute, but any time from 30seconds is fine.

To release the pose, gently exhale and roll the spine towards the floor.

Therapeutic Applications

Relieves constipation.

Helps to relieve the menstrual cramps and reduces symptoms of menopause

Therapeutic for respiratory diseases like asthma and sinusitis

Therapeutic for osteoporosis and helps to reduce high blood pressure.

Precautions

People suffering from neck and back injuries should avoid doing this pose.

Noose Pose

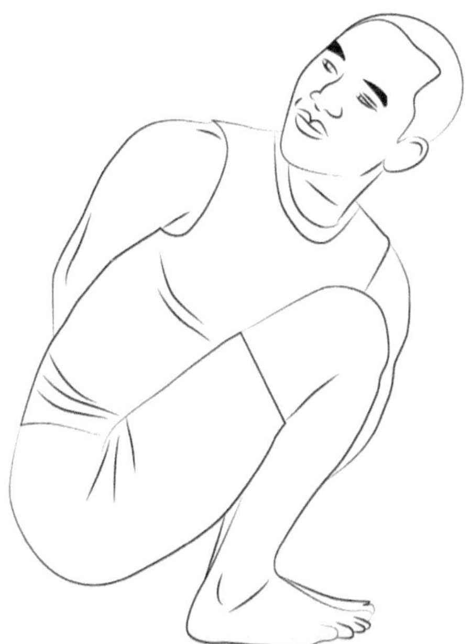

This also known as the Pasasana and is one of the highly referred yoga routines. It is a seated pose and belongs in the intermediate to advanced category that also involves

squatting, bending and twisting of the body at the same time. It helps with trunk flexibility, improves circulation around the backbone and improves nerve health. It also has beneficial effects on the abdominal organs.

Organs

- Feet and ankles
- Abdomen
- Chest and shoulders
- Spine

Benefits

The pasasana stretches and strengthens the ankle

It stretches the spine, groins and thighs.

Stimulates abdominal organs and improves digestion.

Enhances elimination of waste from the body

It opens up the chest and shoulders

It helps to improve posture.

Beginners Tips

Due to the fairly advanced nature of this pose, beginners are generally advised to try a simpler variation of this sequence which involves sanding close to the wall and using the wall as a prop.

Beginners can also use a chair before graduating to using the wall as a prop.

Steps

Begin this pose by standing in the mountain pose (Tadasana). Then bend the knees to assume the position of a complete squat such that the buttocks are close to the heels and the torso is pressed against the thighs. If it is difficult to squat completely with the heels flat on the ground, place a sandbag or a folded blanket below the heels.

Next, swing the knees slightly to the left and while exhaling, twist the torso towards the right side. Extend the left arm and bring its upper part to the outer side of the right knee.

Turn the palm downwards and bend the elbow. Then wrap your forearm around the right shin.

Extend your right arm then sweep it around and towards the back to catch the left wrist. A strap could be used to close the gap in case of difficulty with this step.

Press the knee and arm/shoulder firmly into each other and use this pressure to increase the twist further and lengthen the left side of the torso sliding it atop the thighs.

While inhaling, lift the sternum and lengthen it out through the top of your head then exhale while twisting the body a bit more leading with the left ribs.

Stay in this pose for about 5 slow breaths and release twist.

Repeat for the opposite side

Therapeutic Applications

Relieves back, shoulder and neck tension

Helps with menstrual cramps, flatulence and indigestion

Has a therapeutic advantage in asthma.

Precautions

People with knee and lower back injuries should avoid this asana

In case of herniated disc, do not perform this pose.

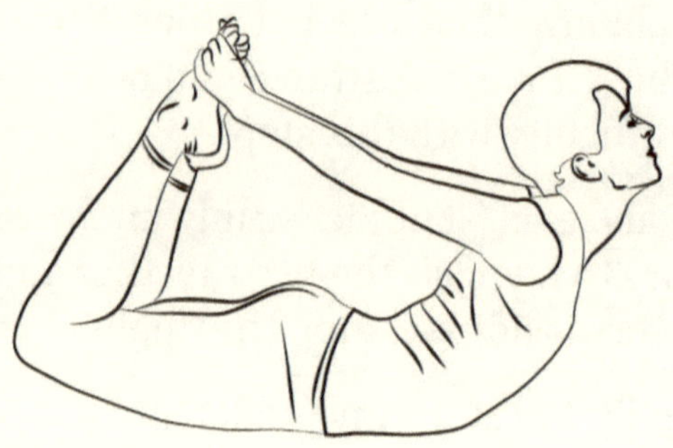

The bow pose is also known as the Dhanurasana and is a direct translation from the Sanskrit word Dhanus which means bow. It is so named because the final posture in this pose assumes the shape of a bow with the chest, abdomen and hips representing the curve of the bow while the arms represent the string. This pose strengthens the abdomen, chest and deep flexors of the hips.

Organs

> Abdomen
> Chest
> Hips
> Thighs

Benefits

This Pose helps to improve posture.

It stretches the whole front of the body, hip region, abdomen, chest and throat.

It also stimulates organs of the abdomen.

It strengthens the back muscles.

Beginners Tips

A rolled-up blanket can be put under the thighs to give it a slight boost if it is difficult to lift the thighs away from the floor.

If it is difficult to reach the feet with the hands, straps can be used, making sure that the arms are fully extended.

Steps

This pose begins with lying flat on the belly with both arms by either side with the palms facing upwards.

Then slowly, while exhaling, raise both legs at the knee bringing the heels as close as possible to the buttocks.

Then take both feet, one in each hand, making sure to grab them at the ankles and not the toes. The knees shouldn't be wider than the width of the hips and they should be kept that way for the duration of the pose.

Inhale while you slowly raise your head and torso, and at the same time lift your heels away from your buttocks. This would arch the back and allow the abdomen to bear the weight of the body. Then inhale slowly again and push the heels further away from the buttocks. Bring the shoulder blades together as you do this as it will open up the heart.

Hold this pose for approximately 30seconds or for as long as you can.

Then slowly, while exhaling, release yourself slowly by lowering you torso to the ground till your chin touches the floor then release your legs from your arms as you return to the starting position.

Lie in this pose for a few breath cycles and repeat if desired.

Therapeutic Applications

Relieves constipation.

Alleviates respiratory symptoms.

Reduces menstrual discomfort and mild back ache.

Helps with fatigue and anxiety.

Precautions

People with severe low back pain, serious neck injury, migraine, sleeplessness and unstable blood pressure should seek medical advice before performing this pose.

Cow Pose

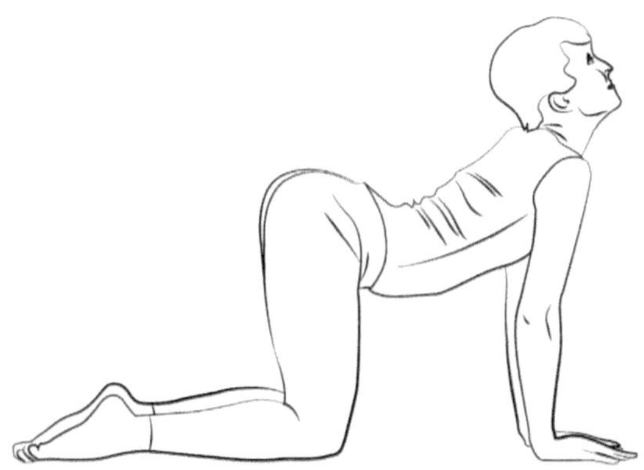

The cow face pose is known as the Gomukhasana in Sanskrit. It is a seated pose that opens up the chest to facilitate deep breathing. It also stretches the arms and shoulders to relieve tension from the shoulders and helps to eliminate rounded shoulders. It is called the cow face pose because the posture assumed at the end resembles the face of a cow.

Organs

- ➤ Chest
- ➤ Lungs
- ➤ Shoulders
- ➤ Arms

Beginners Tips

Beginners can use a folded a blanket to lift the sitting bones off the floor to make it easier for the knees to stack on top of each other evenly

Benefits

Stretches the arms and shoulders

This pose helps to improve posture.

Teaches deep breathing.

Steps

Begin this procedure by assuming the staff pose.

Then bend your knees and keep the feet on the floor. Slide the right left knee under the right knee so that the right knee is stacked on top of the left and bring your right heel close to outside of your left hip. With the right leg on top, tug the right heel in closer to the left hip to bring the heels equidistant from the hips.

Place your palms on the feet.

Sit evenly on sitting bones and point the crown of the head upwards towards the ceiling.

Extend the left arm outwards with the palms facing up, this should roll the shoulders slightly upwards and forward and around the upper back. While exhaling fully, bring the left forearm behind the back and position it in the middle of the back, close to the scapula. The fingers of the left hand should point upwards.

Inhale and stretch the right arm out in front of you, parallel to the floor with the fingers pointing straight. Then with another inhalation, bring it over your head stretched towards the ceiling with the palms facing backwards.

Then bend the right elbow behind the back so that the palm faces the back and the fingers pointing downwards. The elbow should be on the plane between the shoulder blades.

Hook the fingers of the left hand with the right hand and pull the shoulders away from each other. You will feel the stretch in your shoulders and opening of your chest.

Remain in this pose for between 10 and 30 seconds and release by slowly returning to the staff pose.

Repeat steps for the opposite side.

Therapeutic Applications

The cow face pose is therapeutic for common cold.

Opens up the chest and reduces severity and frequency of allergic reactions like sneezing.

Precautions

People with severe problems of the neck and shoulders are advised to avoid this asana.

Extended Puppy Pose

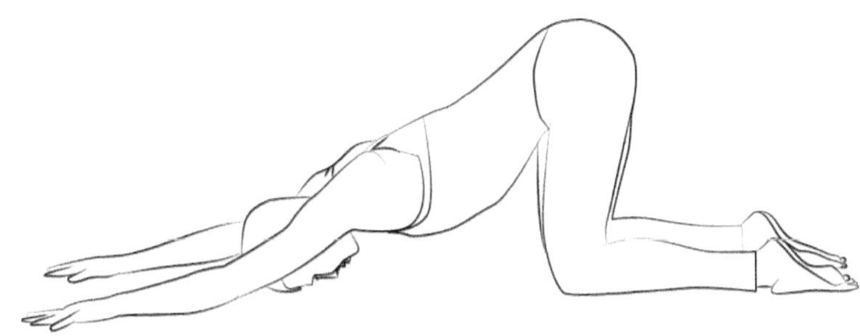

Also known as the Uttana Shisosana, the extended puppy pose is a yoga pose of the forward bend variety. It is regarded as of the simpler and easier forward bends in yoga and such is suitable for beginners. It is not considered a restorative pose but is highly recommended when relaxation of the body and mind is required. It can be incorporated into a lot of other yoga sequences.

Organs

> Chest
> Spine
> Shoulders
> Arms
> Upper back

Benefits

It expands the chest and improves breathing.

It strengthens the hips, upper back and arms.

It refreshes the body.

It stretches the shoulder and spine.

It calms the mind and relieves stress

Beginners Tips

This pose might sometimes prove difficult for a beginner as they often find it difficult to hold this pose for an extended duration. To combat this, as well as support the knees and lower back, a rolled up blanket or a bolster can be placed between the calves and thighs.

Steps

Begin this pose by staying on all fours with the hands and knees like a table where the back is the surface of the table. Make sure the wrists are aligned with the shoulders and the knees positioned directly below the hips.

Now, using the hands, walk forwards slowly and lower the chest towards the floor.

While exhaling, slide the buttocks downward towards the feet till it reaches halfway to the feet. While doing this, make sure that the arms are straight and hands are still on the floor.

Male sure that the elbows aren't touching the ground and the forearms should not be hitting the ground.

Now, slowly move the head forward until your forehead touches the ground. Arch your back towards the floor while doing this, keeping s slight curve in the lower back. Your arms should now be resting on the floor in front of you. Press the hands down and stretch through the arms while pulling the hips backwards to feel a nice long stretch in the spine.

Next, push your hips back and stretch your spine, lengthening it.

Breather deeply in this posture and retain this position for between 30seconds to 1minute

Therapeutic Applications

This asana stretches the spine and shoulders

It is also very beneficial in people who have difficulty sleeping

It helps to relieve tension and long standing stress.

Precautions

People who have knee injuries are advised to stay away from this pose.

This pose is best practiced under supervision by an experienced yoga instructor.

Hare Pose

The hare pose is also known as the Shashankasana in Sanskrit. The final posture in this pose resembles a sitting hare, and that's where it derives its name from. This pose is very helpful in calming the nerves and providing a feeling of tranquility. It also brings a total relief to the spine as well as improves memory and concentration.

Organs

- ➤ Chest
- ➤ Abdomen
- ➤ Adrenals
- ➤ Spine

Benefits

It improves breathing.

It improves heart function and circulation to vital organs in the body.

It strengthens multiple muscles like those of the back, buttocks and pelvis.

It massages internal organs of the abdomen improving function of organs like the liver and spleen.

It is said to have some benefits to the reproductive organs.

It helps in better extension and flexion and flexion of joints.

Beginners Tips

Beginners preferably should perform this pose after being comfortable with the half head stand.

When releasing yourself from this pose, end with a slow inhalation as there is a possibility of light headedness.

Steps

To start this pose, first assume the diamond pose with both palms placed firmly on the knees. The neck and backbone should be kept straight.

Close your eyes and begin to focus on your breathing as well as your body. It is okay during the early stages to practice it with the eyes open but as you progress, endeavor to do it with the eyes closed as that is the ideal posturing.

Take a deep breath and bring the hands above the shoulder, taking care not to allow the elbows to bend. Maintain an equal distance between the arms with the fingers raised and pointing upwards.

Exhaling slowly, reach down to touch the ground with the head and both hands. The hands should touch the ground with the palms facing downwards and only the fingertips on the ground. Relax when the forehead and fingers touch the ground. Your chest and abdomen should be resting on your thighs.

Let the upper trunk relax and remain in this position for a while with the arms kept straight and the neck also straight between both arms.

To release yourself from this pose, exhale slowly while placing the palms on the knees and inhale as you stand up to prevent lightheadedness. The cycle may be repeated up to 5 times.

Therapeutic Applications

Helps with sexual dysfunction

Relaxes the nervous system

It relieves the pain of sciatica.

Precautions

People with vertigo should perform this pose.

Those with slipped disc are also advised to stay away.

It is not healthy for people with hypertension and heart related diseases.

Easy Pose

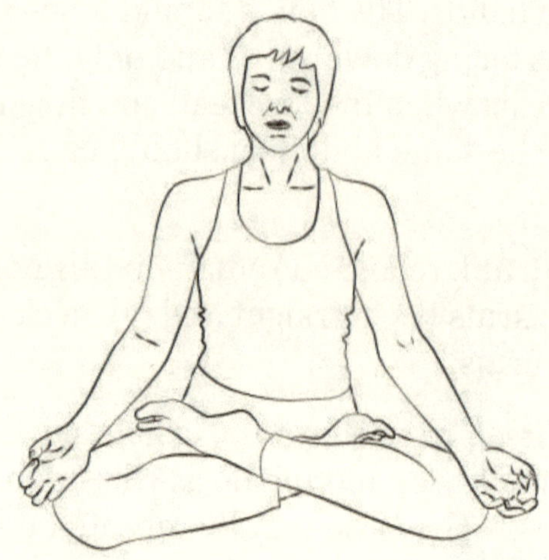

This pose is known in Sanskrit as the Sukhasana. It is called the easy pose, mainly because it is one of the most popular yoga poses and is regarded as the easiest to perform. Beginners are generally advised to start with this pose as it is the entry to the more advanced yoga poses. It is a meditative pose and which helps a in soothing the mind.

Organs

- ➤ Chest
- ➤ Brain
- ➤ Spine
- ➤ Hips

Benefits

It broadens the chest and shoulders.

Calms the brain.

Removes stress, mental exhaustion and anxiety.

Improves states of tranquillity and serenity.

Promotes inner peace.

Lengthens the spine and straightens the back, improving posture.

Reduces fatigue

Stretches the ankles and knees.

Beginners Tips

An individual new to yoga might use a yoga block or a padded cushion for extra comfort.

Sit close to a wall, slightly closer than the width of the cushion or yoga block so that you can wedge either between the wall and your scapular.

Place a folded blanket under the hip bones and knees for added comfort.

Steps

To begin, fold a thick blanket and place on the floor so that it form a thick flat base that can be sat on. It should be about 6 inches in height.

Sit on the edge of this folded blanket with both legs stretched out in front.

Next, cross the legs at the shin and begin to widen the knees so that each foot slips beneath the opposite knee. Then bend the knees and fold the legs inwards towards the trunk.

Relax both feet so that the outer edges rest on the floor and the inner arches are settled just below the shin on the opposite side.

If there is a triangle, formed by the two thighs and crossed shins, then you have gotten the basic leg fold of the Sukhasana. There should be a comfortable gap between the pelvis and the feet.

Sit with your pelvis in a neutral position. To attain a neutral position, lift your sitting bones a bit using your hands, stay there for a breath or two to then slowly lower yourself into the sitting position making sure that the coccyx and pelvis are equidistant from the floor.

Place both palms on the knees with the tailbone stretched towards the floor.

Remain in this pose for as long as it is comfortable and release the pose in reverse order.

If this pose is done often, it is advisable to interchange the position of the legs.

Therapeutic Applications

Recommended for those suffering extreme stress.

Helpful in relieving hip tension.

Precautions

People with knee and hip injuries as well as spinal disc problems should avoid this pose.

Crocodile Pose

Also known as the Makarasana, the crocodile pose stretches and strengthens the back, legs and buttocks as well the back of the arms. This makes it a great asana for all round stretching of the body. It is a deceptively simple pose that is greatly useful in improving posture. The principal focus of this pose is to relieve the strain brought about by other poses, and it is generally regarded as a restorative yoga pose.

Organs

- ➢ Abdomen
- ➢ Chest
- ➢ Legs
- ➢ Arms
- ➢ Pelvis

Benefits

It lengthens the spine and helps to relieve lower back compression.

Harmonises the body and mind

It has an anti-stress effect

It revives physiological balance

Enhances witness-like attitude which helps with meditation.

Beginners Tips

Because of the calming nature of this pose, it is not uncommon for beginners to fall asleep. It is important to remain awake during this pose.

Steps

Start this pose by lying flat on the abdomen with both arms flat on each side and the feet stretched out and slightly apart.

The forehead should be resting on the floor.

Now bring both arms towards the forehead from the side with only a slight raise from the floor. Do not move your body as you do this and move the hands slowly, imagining there is a weight pressing against it from above.

Let both palms come to rest beneath the forehead such that one palm is on the top of the other. You can now adjust your hands slightly forwards or backwards to a position comfortable for your head.

Next, stretch both legs and move them slowly away from each other such that the feet are pointed away from the body.

Remain in this position and focus on the breathing, you should feel a pleasurable pressure on the abdomen as it moves with the breathing.

This pose can be held for as long as possible as it is a restorative pose.

When done, release yourself by slowly returning to the starting position.

Therapeutic Applications

This pose relieves digestive symptoms like flatulence, indigestion and constipation.

It is also helpful in controlling high blood pressure.

It relieves back pain and fatigue.

Relieves headaches and neck pains.

Precautions

Avoid this pose in a case of serious back injury.

In case of neck injury, a folded blanket can be used to support the head, and the head should be in a neutral position.

Individuals with stomach ulcer should seek medical attention before performing this pose.

Garland Pose

It is also known as the Malasana and although it is a squatting pose, it is classified as a standing yoga pose. It may also be referred to as a transition pose as it is often placed in the middle of yoga sessions due to its relative simplicity with just enough to keep the body's rhythm going while taking a break. The pose helps to strengthen muscles of the feet and is recommended for athletes. It also improves the digestive system.

Organs

- Ankles
- Abdomen
- Legs
- Knees

Benefits

It tones the belly

It strengthens and stretches the ankles as well as the groin and back.

It improves digestion leading to more efficient expulsion of waste.

Beginners Tips

In case of difficulty squatting, sit on the front edge of a chair with both thighs in front and at right angle to the trunk. With the heels on the floor and slightly ahead of the knees, lean the trunk forward between the thighs to between the knees. This can be done until full flexibility is achieved and the pose can be done as intended.

Steps

Begin this pose by squatting on the floor, keeping the feet as close together as possible. The feet should be flat on the floor with the heels touching the ground. The heels should also be facing forward on the floor. In case of difficulty keeping the heels completely flat, a folded blanket may be used to support the feet and the base.

Next, gently separate the thighs. They should be separated wide enough for the torso to comfortable slip into. After your torso has fit in snugly, join your hands in a salutation seal (Anjali Mudra) and press your elbows against the inner surface of your knees. This will lengthen the front torso further.

After that has been done, press the inner thighs against the trunk. Then put the arms beyond the folded legs and press the shins into the armpits.

To help the torso stretch and lengthen further, reach your arms forward, then swing them put to the sides and fix your shins into your armpit. Then press the finger tips to the floor or reach around to clasp the back of the heels.

Hold this pose for between 30seconds to 1minute.

Inhale slowly as you stand up from this pose, stretching the knees and standing into Uttanasana.

Therapeutic Applications

It is recommended for pregnant women as it helps to widen the hips making it an ideal preparation for labor.

This pose has been known to bring about induction of labor.

Precautions

People with lower back or knee injuries should avoid this pose.

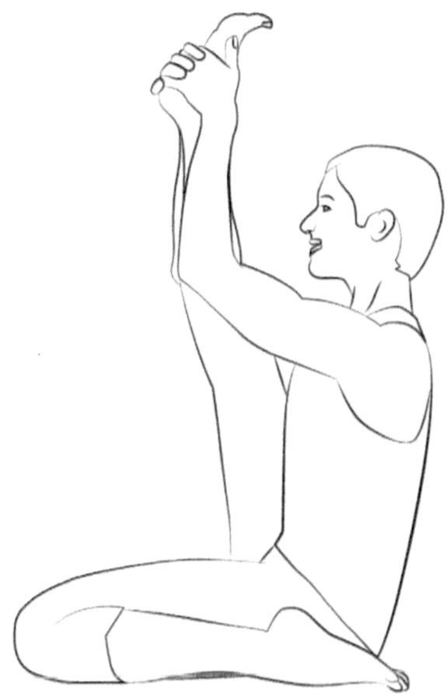

It is also known as the Krounchasana and is a seated yoga pose in the advanced category. It is precisely a stretch while seated that helps exercise the hamstrings and calves, and the knees and hamstrings need to be very supple to accomplish this pose. It is an elegant pose that strengthens the core muscles and stretches the back of the legs.

Organs

- ➢ Leg
- ➢ Feet
- ➢ Chest
- ➢ Abdomen

Benefits

In the legs, it increases the strength of the muscles and improves flexibility of the joints.

It stimulates abdominal and chest organs.

It stretches the ankle, the arches of the feet and the Achilles' heel.

Beginners Tips

Most beginners will have difficulty with the down leg in Ardha Virasana so it is preferable to start with the down leg in the pose for Janu Sirsasana

Steps

Begin by sitting on the floor with the legs stretched out in front in the Dandasana.

Bend the right knee in front of you and place the foot on the floor, just in front of the sitting bone.

Maintain this balance while you sit straight up so that all of you body weight now rests on the sitting bones. Try as much as possible to divide the body weight equally between the two sitting bones.

Then, bend your left knee towards the back so that the left foot rests flat on the floor just in front of the sitting bone. This is the Ardha Virasana.

Place the right arm against the inside of the right leg so that the shoulder is pressing against the inner knee, then cross your hand in front of the right ankle to grasp the outside of the right foot. With the left hand, grasp the inside of the right foot with the left hand.

Leaning back slightly, but keeping the torso long, firm the shoulders blades against the back to maintain the lift of the chest.

While inhaling, raise the legs diagonally as high as possible. Then move the chin towards the knee while keeping the back straight and extended.

Hold this pose for about 30 seconds before lowering the leg slowly.

Repeat all the steps with the opposite leg

Therapeutic Applications

It stretches the arches of the foot which is therapeutic for flat feet.

Its effect on abdominal organs helps with flatulence.

Precautions

It is unsafe to practice this pose during menstruation

In case of knee or ankle problems, avoid the Adhar Virasana part of this pose.

Because of the advanced nature of this asana, it is advised that beginners stay away from it or an experienced yoga instructor should be present if it has to be done.

Corn Tree Pose

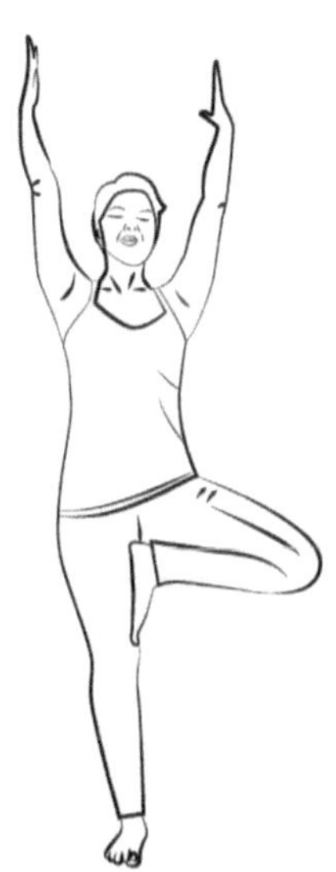

This pose is known as the in Sanskrit. It is a standing pose and is one of the most popular of its kind for beginners. It is relatively easy to perform and thus is ideal for people who have just taken up yoga. It is a stretching pose that benefit the ankles, thighs and pelvic floor muscles. It is generally used for warm up before moving on to harder poses.

Organs

- ➤ Ankles
- ➤ Thighs
- ➤ Pelvis
- ➤ Legs

Benefits

Stretches the whole body.

Strengthens the legs, ankles and feet.

Increases flexibility of the hips and knees.

Beginners Tips

For beginners, the raised foot might keep sliding down the inner thigh. To prevent this from happening, fold a sticky yoga mat and insert it between the foot and thigh. This should provide enough friction to prevent the food from sliding down.

Steps

Stand straight with both arms high up in the air such that you can feel a stretch in both arms on the trunk.

Plant the left leg firmly on the floor and shift the weight of the body slowly unto it.

While inhaling deeply, bend the right knee and with the right hand, hold the right ankle and draw the foot upwards away from the ground. Then place the sole of the right foot on the inner area of the left groin. The toes of the right foot must remain pointed towards the floor.

Straighten the pelvis and ensure that its center is directly over the left foot.

Rest both hands on the rim of the pelvis making sure that the pelvis is in a neutral position with the pelvic rim parallel to the floor.

Stretch the torso and lengthen the coccyx, then press the right foot into the left thigh and resist the pressure with the outer part of the left leg.

Place both hands in the Anjali mudra posture in front of the chest. Remain in this pose for between 30minutes to 1hour while starring at a fixed spot on the ground 4 or 5 feet away.

Release yourself from this pose by slowly unfolding while exhaling and coming back to the Tadasana.

Therapeutic Applications

It is ideal for people suffering from sciatica and lower back pain

Precautions

It is best avoided by people who have migraines and people with insomnia.

People with low blood pressure should not perform this pose.

Raising the arms for a long time in people with high blood pressure can lead to cardiac arrest so it is best avoided by hypertensive people.

Yoga Poses By Anatomical Focus

Yoga Poses For Brain

Corpse Pose:

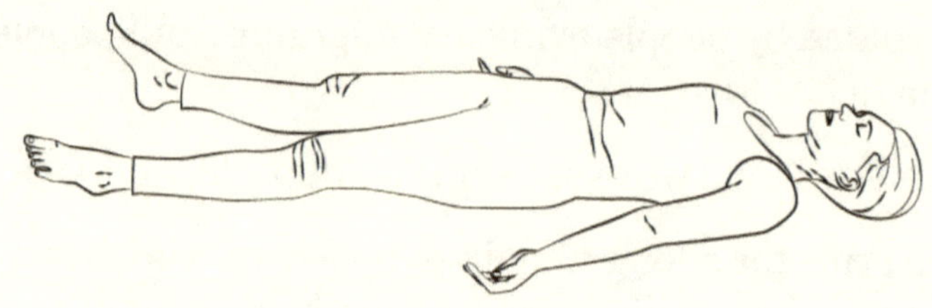

Corpse Pose, is also known as Shavasana in Sanskrit, where the meaning of Shava is corpse and Asana means pose. The reason why it is called as corpse pose is that because this asana looks like a dead body. This pose is generally practiced at the end of the yoga session to get some relaxation.

Organs:

> Heart
> It basically focuses on complete body.

Benefits:

- ➤ It helps in reducing blood pressure.
- ➤ It helps in rejuvenating body and mind.
- ➤ It helps in reducing stress and anxiety.
- ➤ It lessens the tensions and unwanted thoughts from our mind.
- ➤ It helps in relaxing nervous system also.
- ➤ It is also helpful for insomnia.
- ➤ It improves the functioning of brain and also improves heart problems.

Beginner's Tip:

Take 2 sandbags of 10 pounds each and put one across each top thigh, it should be parallel to the groin's crease. And now visualize that both the heads of thigh bones are falling away from the weight, into the floor.

Steps:

1. Lie flat on your back on floor.
2. Now spread your legs one to two feet apart, your heels facing each other and keep your arms also a little apart from your body, palms facing upward.
3. Now get relaxed. And close your eyes.
4. From the toes to fingers to the head scan every part of the body. And try to release and relax any parts that you find.
5. Start breathing slowly and deeply. And release all control of the mind and body.
6. With every breath try to relax yourself more and more.
7. Drop all your thoughts of urgency and feel your breath and body and get relax.
8. But make sure that you don't fall asleep.
9. After 10-15 minutes, when you feel completely relaxed then slowly turn or roll on to your right side keeping your eyes close.
10. Lie in this position for 1-2minute.
11. Now from your right hand take support and slowly sit up in a seated pose.
12. Keep your eyes closed; take few deep breaths in and out. And then gently open your eyes.

Therapeutic Applications:

It helps in relieving from stress and fatigue.
It helps in the treatment of heart problems.
It helps to cure high blood pressure and insomnia.

Precautions:

Don't perform this pose if you have lower back problems or back injuries.
Do not sleep while doing this as it will prevent the decrement in nerve impulses.
Pregnant women should make use of cushions for raising their head and chest.
For everyone, it is an advice to consult a physician or doctor before performing this pose.

Dolphin Pose:

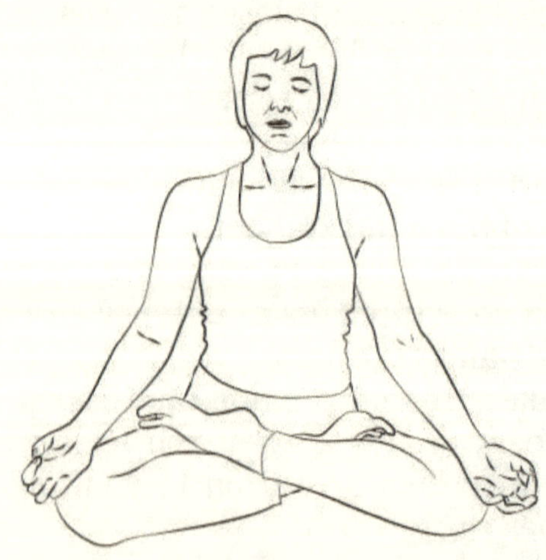

This pose is very helpful in healing many of ailments like asthma, insomnia etc.

Organs:

> ➢ Shoulders
> ➢ Arms
> ➢ legs

Benefits:

> ➢ It helps in stretching shoulders, arms, upper body and legs.
> ➢ It helps in improving digestive system.
> ➢ It helps in relieving the symptoms of menopause.
> ➢ It also reduces stress and depression with calming down your mind.
> ➢ It also helps in reducing headache and symptoms of insomnia.
> ➢ It helps in increasing memory power as well as the levels of concentration.
> ➢ It helps in getting relief from sinus and asthma.

Beginner's Tip:

If your back is bending or arching, even if you have kept your legs straight, then slightly bend your knees so that you can keep the extension in your spine.

Steps:

1. First, come in Table position i.e., on your hands and knees.
2. Keep your forearms on the floor parallel to each other, palms facing down. And your elbow should be directly under your shoulders, and your knees below your hips.
3. While coming in this position press your hands and lower your forearms into the floor.
4. Now slowly exhale and curl your toes under.
5. Now raise your knees off the floor and keep your knees bent as to find length in your spine.
6. Move your hips up towards the ceiling, and lift the sit bones towards the wall at your back.

7. Lift your inner legs up into the groin and press your forearms into the floor.
8. Keep your shoulder blades down in a firm position while maintaining gap between them.
9. Try to hold this pose for few seconds.
10. Now exhale slowly, bend your knees and come back to the floor.

Therapeutic Applications:

It helps in treatment of high blood pressure.
It also helps to cure sciatica and asthma.

Precautions:

Do not perform this pose if you have back pain or any injury.
Avoid this pose if you have high blood pressure.
Don't practice this pose if recently had a shoulder or arm injury.
Avoid this if you have neck pain or neck injury.
For pregnant women and people who are suffering from some medical issues must consult their doctor to perform this pose.

Lotus Pose:

In Sanskrit, it is named as Padmasana. It is derived from the words, Padma which means lotus and Asana means seat. While performing this pose, our shape appears like a lotus, this is also one of the reasons why it is called lotus pose. This pose can be practised by everyone.

Organs:

> Spine
> Thighs
> Ankles

Benefits:

> It helps in reducing stress and calming down the brain.

- ➢ It helps in relieving from pain of sciatica.
- ➢ It also helps in improving body posture.
- ➢ It increases blood circulation in body.
- ➢ It helps in stretching thighs, ankles, calf muscles and spine.
- ➢ This asana also helps pregnant women in easing childbirth but before performing you please consult your gynecologist.
- ➢ It also increases the concentration levels.
- ➢ It helps in digestion as well.

Beginner's Tip:

While doing this pose, take care of your knees. And make sure that you rotate from your hip and not from your knee.
Try to practice preparatory pose, when you hold your leg in the arm and try to open your hips.

Steps:

1. Sit on the ground and stretch your legs straight outside in front of you.
2. Bend your right side knee and keep it on your left thighs.
3. In this position, the sole of the feet should point upward and heel should be close to the abdomen.
4. Now bend your left side knee and keep it on your right thighs in the same position as earlier.
5. Now your both legs are crossed and feet are placed on opposite thighs.
6. Keep your backside of the hands on the knees in mudra position that means your thumb and first finger should be touching.
7. Keep your Spine long and straight and also your head in straight position.
8. Now breathe slowly in and out.

Therapeutic Application:

It helps in the treatment of sciatica and menstrual problems.
It helps in improving concentration level.

It also helps in improving the functions of digestive system.

Precautions:

Do not perform this pose if you have sprain in the leg.
Avoid this pose if you are having injury in your ankle.
Don't do this yoga pose if you are suffering from back pain.
Avoid this pose if you recently had knee surgery or if you are having knee injury.
Before performing this pose you may consult your doctor, if you have any medical issues.

Yoga Poses For Pituitary Gland

Wheel Pose:

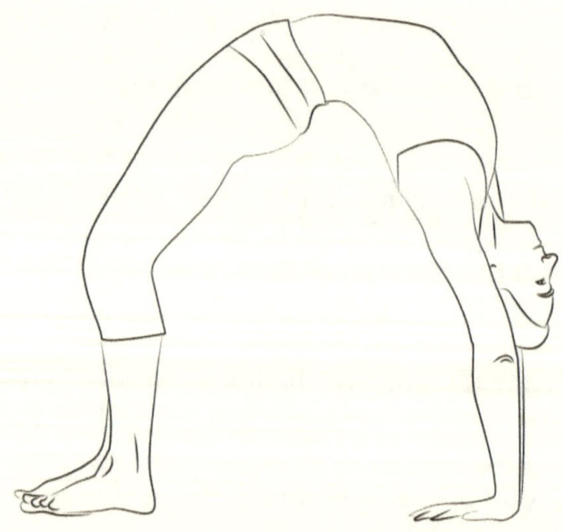

The Sanskrit name of this pose is Urdhva Dhanurasana, where Urdhva means upward, Dhanu means bow and Asana means posture. This is also called Upward Bow Pose. It is one of the backbend poses and it is often practiced at the end of yoga session.

Organs:

> ➢ Shoulders
> ➢ Forearms
> ➢ Legs
> ➢ Chest
> ➢ Lungs

Benefits:

> ➢ It helps in stretching spine, upper back and thighs.
> ➢ It helps in opening the lungs.
> ➢ It also helps in reducing symptoms of asthma.
> ➢ It helps in relieving from depression.
> ➢ It also stretches shoulders and chest.
> ➢ It helps in strengthening arms, wrists, legs and abdomen.

Beginner's Tip:

Beginners should loop a band slightly above the knees and also around the thighs. This will make thighs held at hips width and parallel to each other.

Steps:

1. Lie flat on your back on the floor. And put your arms at your sides.
2. Now bend your knees by keeping your feet aligned to your hips and in a parallel position.
3. Place your heels close to your hips.
4. Now bend your elbows and keep your hands next to your head on the floor.
5. Open your palms wide and your fingers should be pointing towards the shoulders.
6. Try to press your shoulders down in the floor and try to lift your chest and take your tailbone inside. Press down your inner feet.
7. Now inhale while pressing your feet into the floor and try to raise your hips upward towards the ceiling.

8. Contract your hips, thighs, abdominal muscles so that you can support your lower back.
9. Continuously press your hands and feet downwards, while lifting your hips and stomach as much as possible.
10. Hold your breath for some time.
11. And then exhale slowly and come back to the floor.
12. Slide your legs straight on the floor like you are coming to shavasana.

Therapeutic Applications:

It helps in treatment of asthma and osteoporosis.
It also helps in breathing by opening the accessory muscles.

Precautions:

Avoid this pose if you are suffering from low or high blood pressure.
Do not practice it if you are having headaches.
Avoid this pose if you are suffering from diarrhoea.
If you have heart problems, do not perform this pose.
Also avoid this pose in case you have back pain or back injury.
And once consult a physician before doing this.

Pigeon Pose:

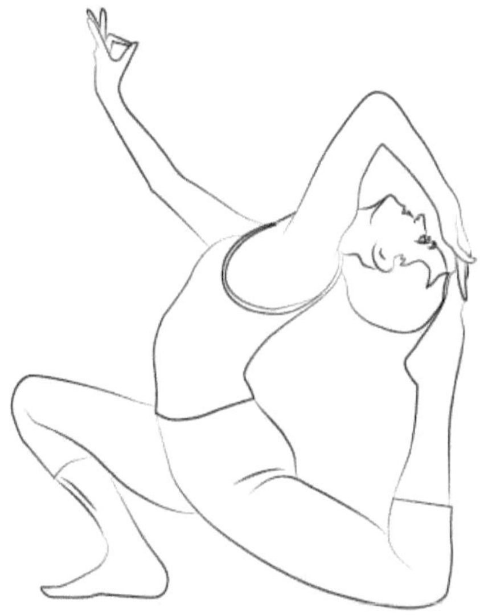

In Sanskrit, we also call this pose as Eka Pada Rajakapotasana, where Eka means one, Pada means foot, Raja means king, Kapota means pigeon and Asana means pose. It helps in opening hips and also increases flexibility.

Organs:

- ➢ Chest
- ➢ Shoulders
- ➢ Abdomen
- ➢ Thighs

Benefits:

- ➢ It helps in stretching thighs and hips.
- ➢ It also helps in urinary disorders.
- ➢ It helps in stimulating internal organs.
- ➢ It helps a lot in opening the hips.
- ➢ It also helps in improving digestive system and reproductive systems.
- ➢ It helps in improving the movement in hip-joints.

Beginner's Tip:

Place your right foot close to your left hip or either keep it below your right buttock as it will make your lower leg parallel to your extended leg.
Make a cushion of your palms and place your forehead on your hands so that you can rest properly.

Steps:

1. Start it by coming in a table position that.
2. Bring your right knee forward and keep it behind your right hand.
3. Try to keep your ankles in front of your left hip and your lower leg should be parallel with the front of the mat.
4. Try to slide your left leg back as much as your hips can allow you to.
5. Place your legs towards each other so that your hips should be in a square position.
6. Now slowly bring yourself down. If you need any support to keep your hips level then you can place something under your right hips.
7. Slowly inhale now and raise your upper body.
8. Come on the tips of your fingers, your hands and shoulders few inches apart.
9. Now place your navel in and your hip bone down and make your chest open.
10. Now while exhaling, move your hands forward on your fingertips and lower your upper body towards the floor.
11. Now rest on your forehead on the ground.
12. Stay in this position and take few breaths.
13. Now exhale slowly and release your hips.

Therapeutic Applications:

It helps in improving digestion.
It helps in improving immunity system.
It also helps in cure of urinary disorders.

Precautions:

Do not perform this pose if you have knee injury.
Avoid doing this if you have problem in your ankles.
Avoid this pose if you have extreme tightness in your hips.
Pregnant women are not advised to practice this yoga pose without consultation.
It will be better if you practice this pose with a yoga trainer.

Upward Facing Two Foot Staff Pose:

In Sanskrit it is called, Dwi Pada Viparita Dandasana, where Dwi means two, Pada means foot, Viparita means inverted, Danda means staff and Asana means pose. The main focus of this pose is to open chest.

Organs:

> Chest
> Kidney
> Shoulders
> Back
> Thighs

Benefits:

> It helps in stretching back muscles, thigh muscles and calf muscles.
> It also massages kidneys and adrenals.
> It helps in toning pelvic region in women.
> It also strengthens back and thighs.
> It strengthens shoulder muscles also.
> It helps in reducing fat from abdomen.
> It helps in opening chest area also.

Beginner's Tip:

For better performance of this yoga pose, make use of yoga mat so that it can provide support to your arms. And it is advised to perform this pose with the help of a yoga guru.

Steps:

1. Lie flat on your back, and put your heels below your knees and keep your feel a little wider.
2. Now bend and keep your palms on the floor just besides your ear. Your fingertips should be towards your shoulders.
3. Stay in this position only and breathe. Focus on your breathing.
4. Now exhale slowly and push your knees in the direction away from your torso.
5. And raise your shoulders, head and your hips above the floor.
6. Straighten your arms while doing this.
7. Move your shoulder blades towards your hip bone.
8. Now let the tip of your head rest on the floor slowly and try to keep your elbows at a distance.
9. Now again exhale and move your one hand towards your ear to hold the back of your head.
10. Allow the weight to be on your forearm.
11. Repeat the same with other hand also.
12. Now exhale deeply and move your chest allowing your head to rise off the floor.
13. Press your heels towards the ground.
14. Hold this position for some time.
15. In the same position allow your feet to be away from your hands, so that your legs can become straight.
16. Now as you have reached to this position, let your head to go back on floor.
17. And allow your middle back to expand more.
18. Now from releasing this pose, make sure you keep your feet are below your knees and your head on the floor. Keep your palms near your ear and your hands below your elbow.
19. Now slowly exhale and then slowly and gently roll down to floor and return to normal position.

Therapeutic Applications:

It helps in the treatment of respiratory diseases.

It also helps to cure the problem of uterus in women.
Precautions:

Avoid this pose if you are having injuries in your back or have lower back pain.
Advised not to perform pose if you have injuries in your wrists and shoulders.
Pregnant women should completely avoid this pose
Do not perform it if you have neck pain or neck injury.
Avoid this yoga pose if you have high blood pressure.
As this is a complicated yoga pose, therefore it is suggested to perform it under the guidance of a yoga guru and also consult your doctor regarding this.

Yoga Poses For Heart

Bridge Pose:

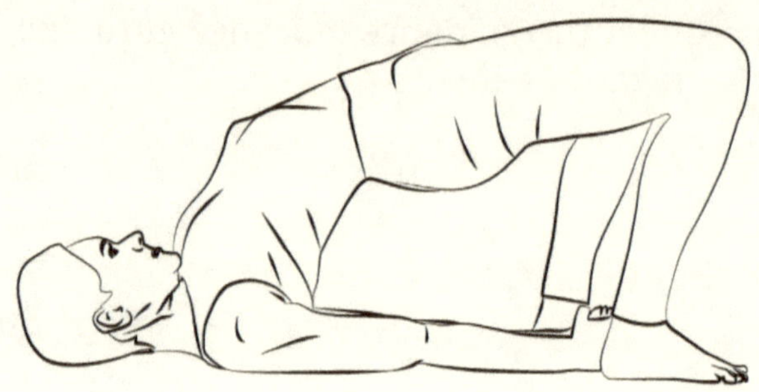

Bridge Pose is also called as Setu Bandhasana in Sanskrit, where Setu means Bridge, Bandh means lock and Asana means posture. It is one of the very important poses as it not only helps for your heart health but it also helps in treatment of other physical illness as well like back pain, neck pain, thyroid problems etc. Basically in this pose we need to bend our back which helps in stretching our thighs as well as in opening our chest.

Organs:

> Chest
> Spine
> Abdominal
> Lungs

Benefits:

- ➢ It helps in opening heart chakras and lungs for better breathing.
- ➢ It helps in stretching out chest, neck, hips and spine.
- ➢ It helps in strengthening the back bones, hips and legs.
- ➢ It reduces stress and insomnia.
- ➢ It also helps in reducing backache and headache.
- ➢ It is also helpful in high blood pressure, sinus, and asthma.
- ➢ Its helps in reducing thyroid problems and relieving from menopause.

Beginner's Tips:

Try stretching your hands towards your feet; it can help you in getting a better pose. Also if you want, you can use Yoga block when you move up.

Steps:

1. Lie on your back (shavasana), with your palms facing down.
2. Take deep breaths so that you can get relaxed.
3. Now bend your knees and keep your feet flat on the floor surface, and bring your heels close to your buttocks or sitting bones. Keep your hips width apart (around 5 to 6 inches).
4. Keep your feet parallel to each other and press your feet as well as your upper arms into the floor. And try to lift your hips upwards towards the ceiling. Take a deep breath while doing this.
5. Try to move your chest towards your chin and not to bring chin towards chest.
6. Support your weight with your arms, feet and shoulders.
7. In this position your thighs should be parallel to the floor and to each other.
8. If you wish you can support your back with your palms.

9. While holding yourself in this position, take couple deep breaths slowly.
10. Try to hold yourself in this position as long as possible.
11. To release from this pose, first bring your feet close towards your hips and then slowly lower your back and release your arms and exhale as you release the pose.

Therapeutic Application:

It can help in opening the sinuses.

Helpful in treatment of osteoporosis.

Precautions:

Avoid doing this yoga pose if you are having back injury or back pain.

Also avoid this pose if you are having neck pain.

Don't move your head right or left while doing this pose.

You should not perform this if you are having knee pain and shoulder injury.

Pregnant women should not perform this pose.

Women should avoid doing this while menstrual cycle.

If you have any medical issues, take advice from a doctor before performing this.

Bow Pose

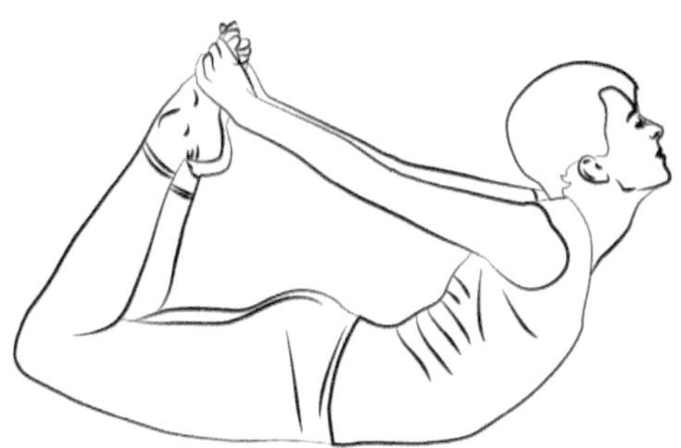

It is also known as Dhanurasana in Sanskrit, where Dhanu means bow and asana means pose. It is named as Bow pose because we form a shape of bow while performing this yoga pose. This yoga pose also have many health benefits including heart health, asthma problem, weight loss etc.

Organs:

- ➤ Chest
- ➤ Thighs
- ➤ Ankles
- ➤ Forearms

Benefits:

- ➤ It is highly effective in weight loss, improving digestion and appetite and cures constipation.
- ➤ It helps in strengthening thighs, chest, ankles, back bones and abdominal.
- ➤ It helps in improving blood circulation.
- ➤ It also helps in curing problems like asthma.

➢ It helps in massaging the heart and improving other body organs like liver, intestine, pancreas etc.
➢ It also helps in reducing stress and depression.

Beginner's Tips:

Starts trying this pose only by lifting your chest up and your thighs and knees on the floor. And also in the beginning, you can take help of belt around your feet to help you reach towards them.

Steps:

1. Lie on your stomach facing downwards, with both your arms on your side.
2. Now take a breath by keeping your forehead on the floor and relax for a while.
3. Start inhaling slowly and bend your legs backward until they almost touch your hips.
4. Now grasp your ankles with your hands.
5. Try to raise your head and torso slowly from the ground.
6. Now your body will be in the form of a bow. And your whole body weight will be on your abdomen.
7. Try to hold this position for as long as you can and slowly take deep breaths.
8. Now for releasing from this pose, put your forehead and torso slowly on the floor and free your ankles from your hand's grasp and lower your feet.
9. Slowly exhale for few seconds while coming back to your original position.

Therapeutic Application:

Helps in relieving menstrual discomfort.

Helps in respiratory ailments.

It is therapeutic for Diabetes and Asthma and Colitis.

Precautions:
People suffering from heart problem or high blood pressure issues should avoid this pose.

One should avoid it if they are having backbone issues or back pain, sciatica, headache and migraine problems.

Do not perform this pose if you are having hernia, ulcer, recent abdominal surgery, appendicitis and colitis.

Pregnant women should completely avoid this. And women in menstrual cycle should also not perform this too.

Never perform this before going to bed at night and also after taking meal.

One who is having a shoulder dislocation earlier should also avoid doing this.

If you are having any health issues, consult a doctor or physician before doing this pose.

Cat Pose

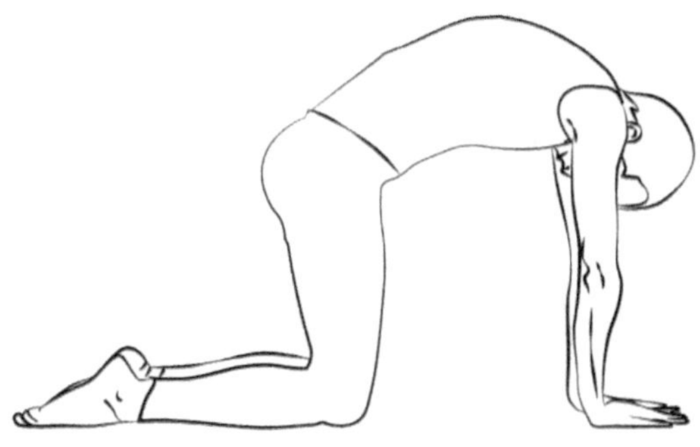

It is also known as Marjariasana in Sanskrit, where Marjari

means cat and asana means posture or pose. It is one of the very common and popular pose that is widely performed. This pose is good for both beginners as well as experts because it won't give you any such injuries or pain. This pose is also known for correcting one's posture.

Organs:

> - Chest
> - Shoulders
> - Wrist
> - Knees

Benefits:

> - It helps in improving the blood circulation and as well as in better digestion.
> - It helps in toning and strengthening arms and abdomen.
> - It helps in stretching back, neck as well as abdominal.
> - It helps in reducing backache and also makes spine flexible.
> - It also helps in relaxing mind.

Beginner's Tips:

Have a friend or someone with you while doing this, so that if you find any difficulty to know whether your back is rounding correctly or not, you can ask your friend to place their hand on your upper back. So it will then activate this part of your body.

Steps:

1. First of all you need to make a pose like a cat, by coming into a table position by putting both your hands and knees on the floor.
2. Keep your knees just below your hips and your hands perpendicular on the ground below your shoulders that means your palms flat on the ground.

3. Now look straight. And make sure that your hands and knees remain in the same position.
4. Now slowly inhale and raise your chin and move your head back.
5. Push your navel towards downward. And raise you hipbone.
6. Now while holding this cat position, take deep breaths.
7. Now as you exhale, move your chin inwards towards your chest and raise your middle back upwards that is towards ceiling by making an arch or rounding back.
8. Try to hold this position for few seconds and after that come back to your initial stage i.e., table position.
9. Do this continuously for 5 to 6 times.

Therapeutic Application:

It helps in releasing the stress by practicing daily.

Precautions:

Do not perform this pose if you are having backbone problems or surgeries.

Avoid this pose if you are having neck pain.

Do not perform this pose if you are having knee pain or wrist injury.

Try to consult a doctor if you are facing any medical issues before performing this pose.

Big Toe Pose

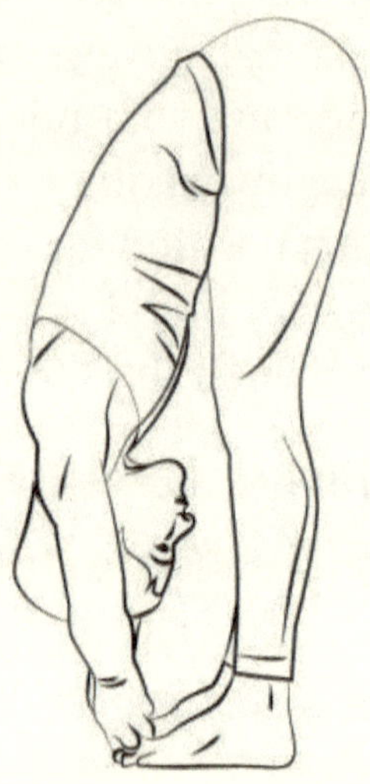

In Sanskrit it is called Padangusthasana, where Pada means foot, Angustha means big toe, and Asana means pose. It is considered as one of the easiest yoga pose. It will benefit whole body from head to toe.

Organs:

- ➢ Thighs
- ➢ Back
- ➢ Spine
- ➢ Arms
- ➢ Liver

Benefits:

- ➢ It helps in regulating the blood pressure and increase the blood circulation in the body.
- ➢ It strengthens your legs, thighs, toes and ankles.

- ➢ It is good for women who are planning to conceive, as it stretches all muscles.
- ➢ It also increases flexibility as it stretches your whole body from head to toe.
- ➢ It helps in improving digestion and also helps in keeping stomach related problems away.
- ➢ It helps in toning kidney, liver, spinal muscles and nerves.
- ➢ It also helps in reducing your mental stress and makes you calm down.
- ➢ It also helps in improving the balance of the body.

Beginner's Tip:

It is important for you to practice this pose with band for few times. Once you get used to it then it will be easier for you to grasp your toes.

Steps:

1. Firstly, stand upright just like mountain pose, keeping your feet parallel to each other and should be at least 6 inches apart from each other.
2. Inhale and keep your legs straight.
3. Now to lift your knee caps outward, contract your thigh muscles.
4. With keeping your legs straight, bend forward to touch your forehead to your knee by moving your head and torso together.
5. After coming to this position, grip your big toes firmly with fingers of each foot.
6. Then try to press your hand with your toes.
7. Now inhale and lift your torso, along with straightening your elbows.
8. Try doing this as long as you can without putting stress to any other organ.
9. Now slowly exhale and release your torso.

10. And again bend towards your toes slightly. And do this posture repeatedly.
11. Now by slowly releasing the band and getting straighten, come back to the starting position.

Therapeutic Applications:

It helps in the treatment of hypertension and high blood pressure.

It also helps to cure osteoporosis.

It helps in reducing headache and insomnia.

Precautions:

Avoid doing this yoga pose if you are having diarrhoea.

One should not perform this while having heavy cold.

Do not perform this pose if you have any sought of back injuries or back pain.

Avoid this yoga pose if you have neck pain.

One should not try doing this to its extreme level if they are having weak ankles.

Always consult a doctor before doing this pose if you have any kind of illness.

Cobra Pose

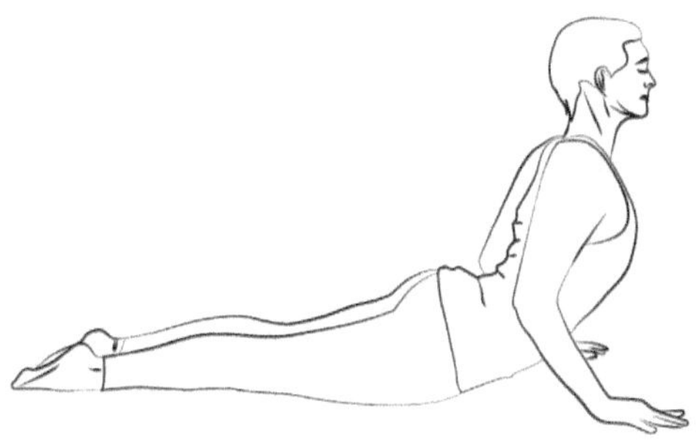

Cobra Pose is also known as Bhujangasana, where Bhujanga refers to serpent or snake and Asana refers to posture. This is really a great yoga pose for those who are suffering from stomach problems, respiratory disorder, and weight gain problems etc. It helps in benefiting our whole body system.

Organs:

- ➤ Spine
- ➤ Neck
- ➤ Abdominal
- ➤ Chest

Benefits:

- ➤ It helps in strengthening shoulders, arms and chest.
- ➤ Blood circulation is also improved with the help of this pose.
- ➤ It also helps in improving the intake and circulation of oxygen especially throughout the pelvic and spinal.
- ➤ It helps in reducing the symptoms of asthma.

- ➤ Removes backache and neck ache.
- ➤ It helps in opening the chest and strengthening central body parts.
- ➤ It also increases the flexibility of spine.
- ➤ It also helps in reducing stress and elevating mood.

Beginner's Tip:

Beginners should take care of their shoulders while doing this and they should try to keep them away from ears and from base of the neck.

Steps:

1. Lie on your stomach, in downward direction.
2. Relax and rest your forehead on the ground and your toes flat on the ground.
3. Put your legs close to each other and your feet and heels touching each other.
4. Keep your palms under below your shoulders.
5. Put your elbows close to torso in a straight position.
6. Now slowly have a deep breath while lifting your head, chest and abdomen and leaving your navel touching the ground.
7. Now your upper body weight will come on your hands and thighs.
8. Try to inhale and exhale as much as you can in this position.
9. Move your head backward as much as you can try to move it and try to stretch yourself.
10. Try to hold your breath for some time in this position.
11. Now while exhaling slowly, bring your chest, abdomen and head to the ground.
12. It will be very effective if you would repeat this cycle 4 to 5 times in a day.

Therapeutic Applications:

It helps in curing gynaecological disorders.

Helps in treatment of sciatica and asthma.

Precautions:
Do not perform this asana if you have ulcer, hernia or if you recently had abdominal surgery.

People who have heart problems should avoid this pose.

Pregnant women should definitely not try this yoga pose.

People who have surgeries like brain, lungs, and spine should not go for this pose.

Women undergoing menstruation should avoid doing this pose.

People suffering from the problem of arthritis and lower back pain are advised not to perform this pose.

Consult your physician before you start practising this pose.

Cow Pose

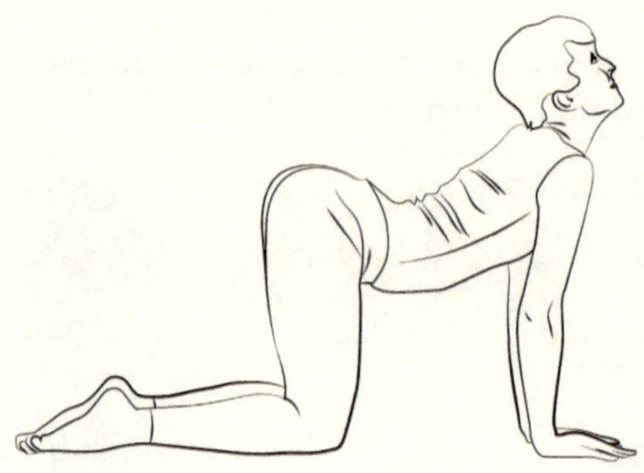

Cow pose is named after its Sanskrit name Bitilasana, where Bitila means cow in Sanskrit and Asana means pose. People who just started learning yoga can try this yoga pose as this pose is not so hard to perform and it also helps in realignment of the body.

Organs:

- ➢ Spine
- ➢ Knee
- ➢ Abdominal
- ➢ Elbow

Benefits:

- ➢ It helps in reducing the pain in your knee joints.
- ➢ It stretches spine, back muscles and neck as well.
- ➢ It also reduces the back pain.
- ➢ It increases the flexibility in spine.
- ➢ It increases the strength of abdominal and also makes arms and elbows strong.

> It also helps in balancing the circulatory system and improves blood flow to chest.
> It reduces the stress and gives relaxation.

Beginner's Tip:

It is advised to the beginners to perform this pose in front of mirror so that they can notice whether their alignment is correct or not.

Steps:

1. First of all, make a pose like a cow, by coming into a tabletop position by putting both your hands and knees on the floor.
2. Keep your knees just below your hips and your hands perpendicular on the ground below your shoulders such that your palm touches flat on the ground.
3. Keep your head in the neutral position and look down towards the floor.
4. Now start inhaling slowly; raise your chest and sitting bones towards the ceiling and drop your stomach towards the ground.
5. Now raise your head and try to look straight forward.
6. Now as you exhale, return back to your neutral position i.e., tabletop position.

Therapeutic Application:
It helps in relieving stress and also in relaxing mind and body.

Precautions:
If you have neck pain or back pain back injuries, please avoid this pose.

Do not perform this yoga pose if you have injuries in your arms or knees.

It is recommended to practice these poses in guidance of a yoga trainer in the initial phases.

Staff Pose

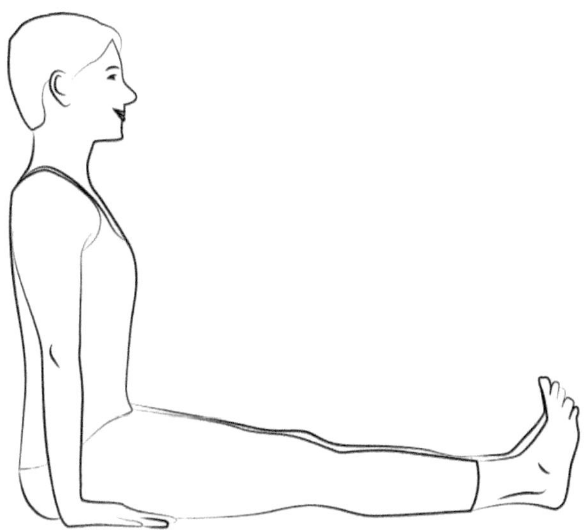

In Sanskrit it is called, Dandasana which is derived from two words that is Danda which means staff and Asana means pose. This pose is also used to prepare different other poses. And it basically focuses on body alignment.

Organs:

> ➤ Thigh
> ➤ Chest
> ➤ Abdomen
> ➤ Lower back

Benefits:

> ➤ It helps in strengthening thigh muscles and calf muscles.
> ➤ It helps in building strength in lower back and abdominal.
> ➤ It helps in stretching chest, abdomen and shoulders.

- ➤ It helps in reducing pain of sciatica.
- ➤ It helps in reducing symptoms of asthma.
- ➤ It also improves body alignment.
- ➤ It helps in relieving stress and improving concentration.
- ➤ It also helps in maintain good body posture.

Beginner's Tip:

As it is a very simple pose, so you will not face much problem in doing this. Just lay one to three sandbags of around 10pounds across the top of your thighs at hip crease to ground your thighs.

Steps:

1. Sit on the ground and stretch out your legs forward in front of you.
2. Your back should not be leaning against anything.
3. Your body should be in perfect vertical alignment.
4. Now press your thighs down in the ground.
5. Rotate your thighs towards each other and try to pull the inner groins towards the sacrum.
6. Now push your heels forward by flexing your ankles.
7. Now try to visualise a flow of energy from your hipbone or pubis going upwards in your torso. It helps you in increasing the length of your back.
8. Now visualise that your hip bone length is growing and is entering into the floor.
9. Imagine as if your spine is your vertical support that helps in controlling all movements.
10. Hold this position for few minutes and exhale slowly.
11. Now with exhaling, slowly release from this position and sit back normally.

Therapeutic Application:

It helps in the treatment of sciatica and asthma.

Precautions:

Avoid doing this if you have back pain or lower back injury.
Do not practice it if you have injury in your wrist.
Consult your doctor or physician before doing this if you have any medical problems.

Bound Angle Pose

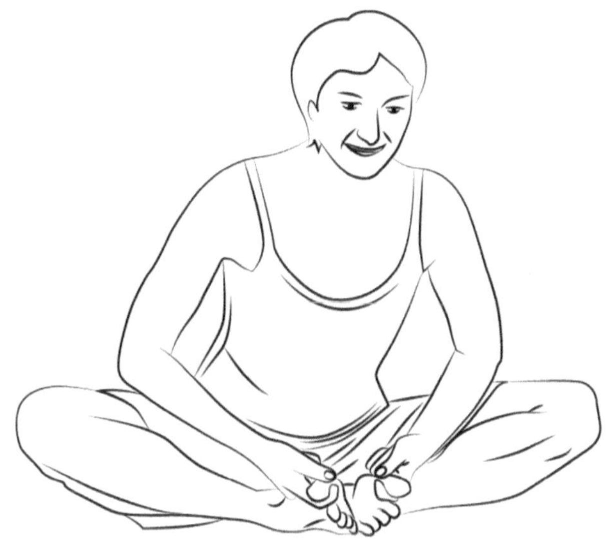

In Sanskrit it is called Baddha Konasana, where Baddha means bound, Kona means angle and Asana means pose. It is given one more name and that is Cobbler's Pose. It is also one of the seated yoga poses and it helps in opening the hips.

Organs:

> Knees
> Ankles
> Thighs
> Pelvic

Benefits:

> It helps in improving blood circulation in the body.
> It also helps in stretching hips, knees and inner thighs.

- ➢ It is very beneficial for pregnant women but it is recommended to consult your gynecologist first before doing this.
- ➢ It also reduces the symptoms of menopause.
- ➢ It also helps in getting relief from frustration and fatigue.

Beginner's Tip:

Sit on a high support, if your knees are high and your back is rounded because it's not easy to lower your knees towards the floor.

Steps:

1. First, sit on the ground and stretch out your legs in front of you straight.
2. Your back should be straight and your hips should be raised. If you want take a blanket and then sit on it.
3. Now bend your knees and pull your feet inward.
4. Keep the soles of the feet together and bring them close to your pelvis as much as you can.
5. Let your knees bent out to the sides.
6. Now release your thigh bones and your groins and bring your knees down for relaxation.
7. Now with your thumb and your first two fingers grasp your big toe.
8. Try to firm your shoulder blades in your upper back so that you can open your heart.
9. Stay in the same position for some time and breathe slowly.
10. To release from this pose slowly lift your knees and straighten your legs.

Therapeutic Applications:

It helps in boosting fertility.
It helps in the treatment of high blood pressure.
It also helps to cure asthma.

Precautions:

Do not practice this pose if you have tight hips.
Avoid this pose if you have lower back problem or back pain.
Avoid this if you have a knee pain or knee injury.
It's always good to practice it with a yoga guru.
Consult your doctor before doing this.

Lord of the Dance Pose

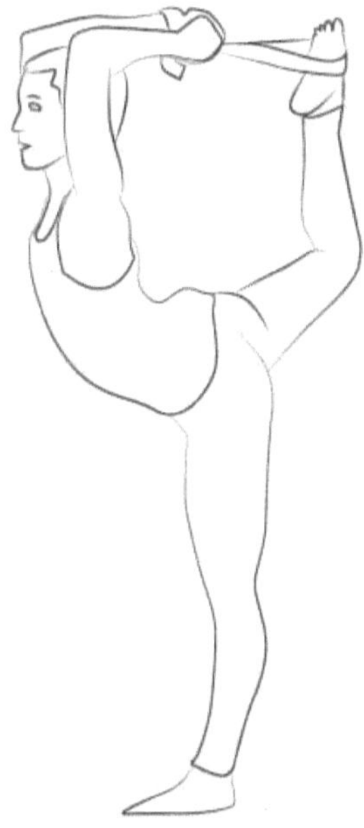

In Sanskrit, it is also named as Natarajasana, where Nata means dance, Raja means king and Asana means pose. This pose has been inspired by the Hindu God Shiva. It is beneficial for chest expansion and strengthening shoulders and thighs muscles.

Organs:

- ➤ Chest
- ➤ Legs
- ➤ Abdomen
- ➤ Ankles
- ➤ Shoulders

Benefits:

> - It helps in weight loss.
> - It helps in stretching thighs and abdomen.
> - It helps in improving digestion.
> - It helps in strengthening chest and legs.
> - It is also good for relieving stress.
> - It also helps in getting good body posture and maintaining balance.

Beginner's Tip:

When you will perform this pose, and will lift your leg then try to keep your lifted ankle flexible so that you do not get cramp in your thigh muscles.

Steps:

1. First stand with your feet together and both your arms by your sides as like we stand in Tadasana or Mountain Pose.
2. Now inhale slowly and bend your right leg backward.
3. Hold your right foot with your right hand by moving your right hand backward.
4. Move your right leg upwards as much as you can.
5. Now extend your left hand straight out in front.
6. Try to hold this position for few seconds while breathing.
7. Now come back to the normal position slowly.
8. Now repeat this with your left leg also.
9. Practice this at least 4 times in a day.

Therapeutic Applications:

It helps in improving and increasing concentration levels.
It also helps in focusing on both mind and body together at one time.

Precautions:

Avoid this pose if you are having low blood pressure problems.

Better to have someone around while practicing this so that if you need help in balancing you can take.
If you have shoulder injuries, avoid this pose.
If you have knee pain then also avoid this.
And consult your doctor before doing this pose.

Poses For Liver

The bridge pose

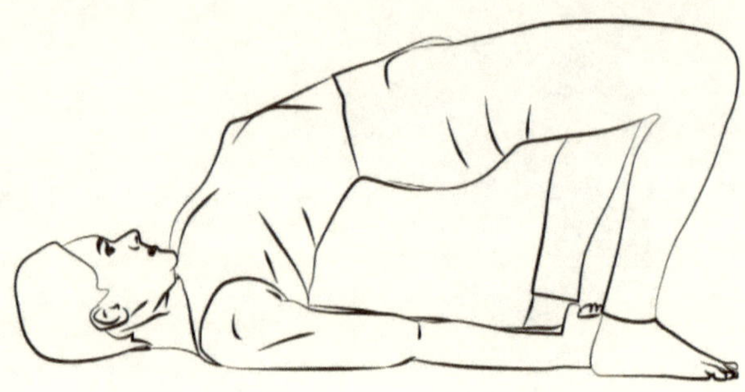

The bridge pose is beneficial to the liver because it strengthens the muscles that strengthen the liver.

Organs

> Back
> Legs
> Arms
> Chest

Benefits

Helps alleviate menopause symptoms

Relieves menstrual cramps

Relieves headaches and backaches

Reduces stress and anxiety

Stimulates abdominal organs such the liver and kidneys

Stretches the neck, spine and chest

Strengthens the legs

Beginner tips

As a beginner, be careful with the shoulders. Do not pull the shoulders away from the ears rapidly or using force- this might injure your neck. It is recommended that you bring the shoulders towards the ears and move the shoulder blades away from your body.

Steps

1. Place a blanket on the floor.
2. Lie in a supine position on the blanket. Place your feet on the floor with your knees bent. Bring the feet together.
3. Breathe out while firmly pressing the feet and hands against the floor. Draw the tailbone towards the ceiling but do not tighten the buttocks. Let the buttocks follow the upward direction of the tailbone.
4. Stop lifting the buttocks once the thighs are nearly parallel to the floor. Position the knees in line with the heels but away from the hips.
5. Maintaining the tailbone behind the knees bring the pubic region closer to the navel.
6. Lift the chin such that you move it away from the sternum. Tighten the shoulder blades and make the arms firm. Move the space between the shoulder blades upwards (the base of the neck).
7. Stay in the position for 1 minute, but 30 seconds are enough.

Therapeutic applications

The bridge pose improves digestion. It is, therefore, widely applied as an alternative to allopathic medicine in treating indigestion problems.

It is incorporated in asthma therapy as it improves inhalation and exhalation.

Other therapeutic applications include osteoporosis therapy, high blood pressure and sinusitis.

Precautions

The bridge pose requires help. Seek the help of a professional yoga trainer. If performed in the wrong way it results in serious neck injury.

The cat pose

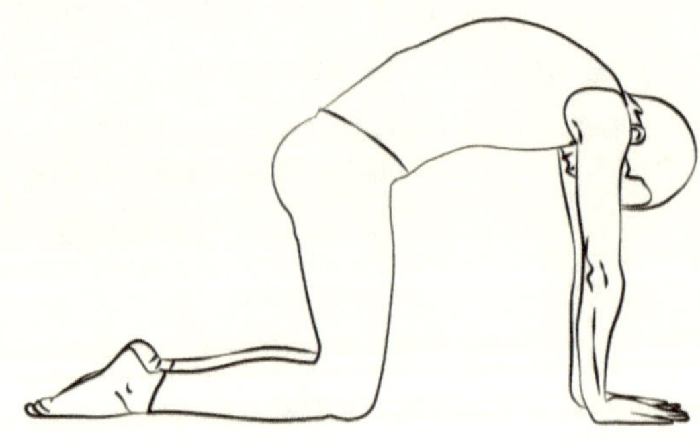

The cat pose is beneficial to the liver since it gently massages and stretches the abdomen. It is a non-complex pose that is easy to learn- a reason it is so popular.

Organs

- ➢ Hands
- ➢ Shoulders
- ➢ Knees
- ➢ Back

➢ Neck

Benefits

Stretches the neck and back

Provides a relaxing massage to the stomach and abdominal organs such as liver and kidneys

Beginners' tips

Beginners may have problems with turning the upper part of the back. The help of a friend or trainer is thus necessary for the pose to be effective. The friend should place their hand on the shoulder blades.

Steps

The cat pose requires keen attention to the steps outlined below. Failing to follow the steps to the letter will reduce the effectiveness of the pose. Keenly following the guidelines is also key to avoiding neck pain and injury. Follow the steps below while performing this pose;

1. Get into a table-top position- this is the position where the hands and knees are on the floor. The pose requires that the knees be in line with the hips. It is mandatory for the shoulders, elbows and wrists to be in line with each other and perfectly perpendicular to the floor. Position the head in a central position with the eyes looking down on the floor.
2. Once you are in position, breathe out while twisting your spine upwards towards the ceiling. Do not shift the position of the hands and knees.
3. Avoid moving your chin towards the chest by gradually lowering it towards the floor.
4. Breathe in as you restore the body to the initial tabletop position.
5. Repeat the procedure as many times as you want.

Therapeutic applications

The pose is used as part of a combination of stress relieving yoga poses

Improves inhalation and exhalation, thus a common recommendation for asthma therapy

Precautions

The pose might hurt your neck if you have an injury. It is thus advisable to keep the neck perpendicular to the torso to avoid pain and\or injury.

The cobra pose

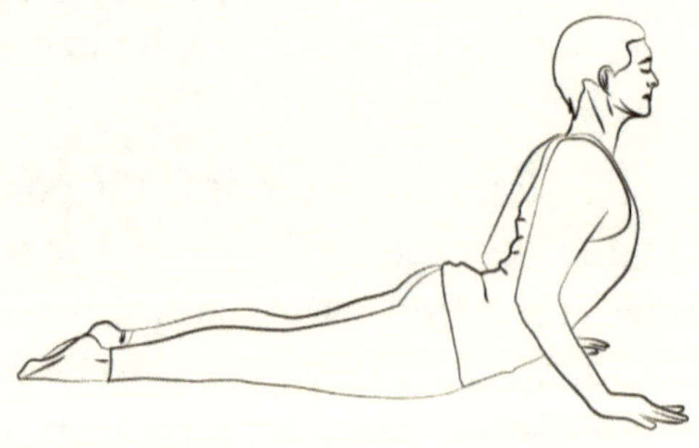

The liver is located in the abdomen, immediately below the chest. The cobra pose opens the chest and stretches the muscles directly above the liver.

Organs

 - ➤ Chest
 - ➤ Arms
 - ➤ Legs
 - ➤ Shoulders

➢ Back

Benefits

Relaxes the sciatic nerve

Strengthens the spine

Makes the buttocks firm

Flexes the chest muscles

Stimulates the heart and lungs

Stimulates the abdomen and its organs including the liver

Stress and fatigue relief

Beginners' tips

The pose involves bending the back. Do not overdo it as it will result in back pain. The essence of yoga is pain relief not the introduction of pain. Yoga specialists recommend that one should first find a level they are comfortable bending from. To find that level one has to take the hands off the floor.

Steps

1. Lie on the ground, your back facing upwards and your abdomen perpendicular to the floor. The top surface of your feet should also be in contact with the floor. Position the hands on the floor in such a way that the elbows face the body.
2. Press the body firmly against the floor.
3. While inhaling, straighten the arms such that they lift the chest away from the floor. Do not lift the chest past a position where you cannot maintain a connection with the pubic region. Draw the pubic area towards the navel and tighten the hips without making the buttocks firm.

4. Push out the ribs by tightening the shoulder blades against the back. The bend in the back should be even throughout the spine.
5. Maintain this position for a maximum of 30 seconds. While exhaling, release the body back to the floor.

Therapeutic applications

Traditionally the cobra pose was used to increase heat in the body and rejuvenate the kundalini.

In the modern day world, the cobra pose is used in asthma therapy. The stretch is good at stimulating the lungs improving inhalation and exhalation. Also improves liver function.

Precautions

The pose is not recommended for pregnant mothers and people with carpal tunnel syndrome. The pose will be very uncomfortable for individuals with back injuries and headaches.

Poses For Bladder

Big toe pose

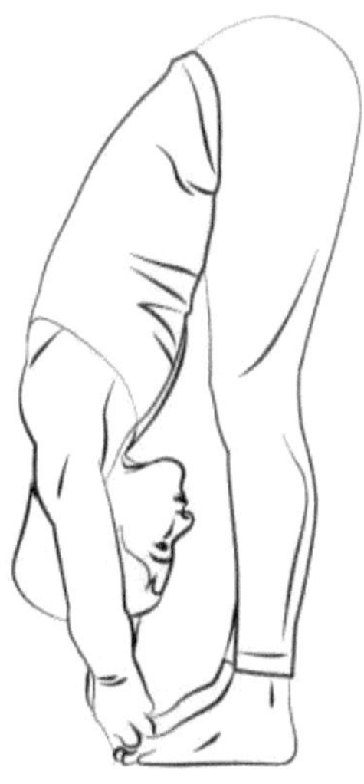

This pose is focusing on the health of bladder. This is a simple pose and you can try it at any time. Make sure you are in easy clothes and start this pose for improved health of bladder. Yoga is all about poses and you can try different poses which are focusing on different parts of the body. This pose is good for health of the body but mainly targets the health of bladder.

Organs

- ➢ Bladder

Benefits

This pose is helpful for increasing the length of hamstrings

Strength of hamstrings is also improved by using this pose

This pose is helpful for improved health of bladder and hamstrings

Beginner tips

You must stand straight for this pose. Then you have to bend the body and go down in such a manner that your body is folded completely. Then you must touch your feet with your hands while keeping your face closer to the legs. Keep your face close to the legs and touch the feet with your hands.

Steps

1. Stand straight in a relaxed mood
2. Inhale and bend towards the ground while keeping the legs straight
3. When you take the face close to the legs then touch the feet and exhale
4. Continue to inhale and exhale while remaining in the position of touching the feet
5. Stay in this position for as long as you feel comfortable before returning and then starting again
6. Normal time for each step is up to one minute

Therapeutic applications

This pose increases length of hamstrings

Strength of hamstrings is also improved through this pose

Your hamstrings will become strong and your balder will become healthy

Precautions

You can try this pose at any time and make sure that you are not imposing extra pressure on the body.

Continue this pose till you feel relaxed and remain safe from stress on muscles and the body.

If you feel stress then stand straight and take some rest

Bound angle pose for health of bladder

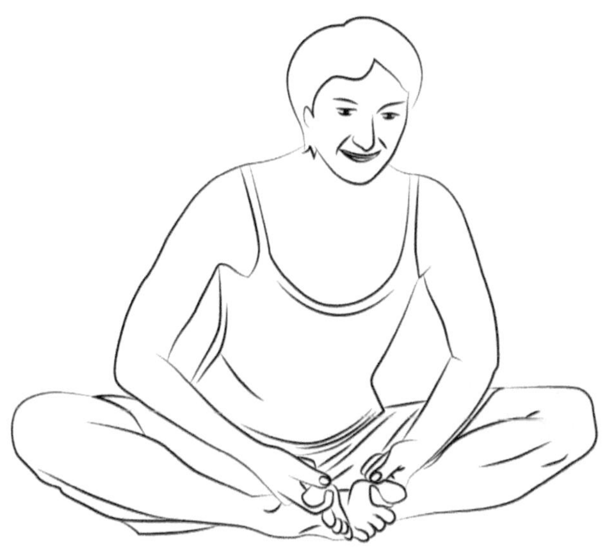

This pose is helpful for those people who remain seated while working or in routine life. This pose is also used as a hip opener. We all sit in routine life and this affects the working of the bladder. This pose is helpful for opening hips and elimination of problems due to excessive sitting. As a result the health and strength of bladder is improved. All poses of yoga are also good for health of the heart.

Organs

- ➢ Bladder
- ➢ Hips

Benefits

This pose helps in relaxation of hips and bladder

Strength of hips and bladder is improved

Beginner tips

You must sit on a straight surface in easy clothes. Then you must hold the big toes of feet with your hands and join the bottom of the feet together. Stay in this position as long as you want.

Steps

1. Sit on a straight surface
2. Fold your legs so that your bottom of feet touch together
3. Hold your big toes of feet with your hands and press the bottom of feet together
4. Remain in this pose for up to one minute and then repeat after taking some rest
5. Your legs must be pressed with thighs in this pose
6. Bottom of the feet must touch each other

Therapeutic applications

Muscles of bladder and hips are relaxed

This pose improves health of bladder and hips

Precautions

Make sure that you are not sitting in this pose for long time and causing stress on the body. When you feel stressed then you must stand straight and continue this pose after relaxation. When you are holding your feet, make sure that your body is in bending position. You must bend a little in the direction of your feet and keep them held while in this pose.

Bridge pose

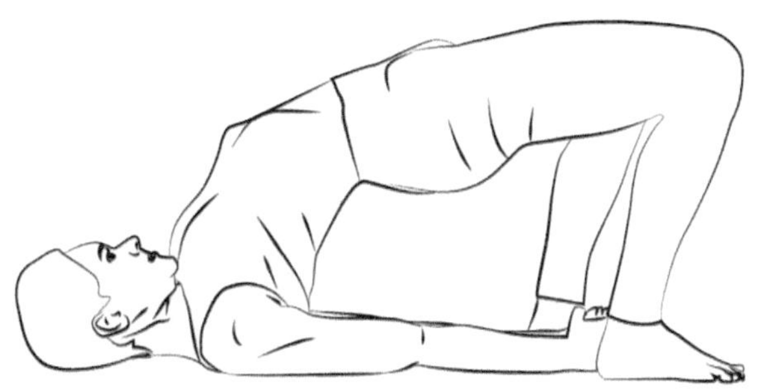

Bridge pose is helpful for increasing strength of bladder. You can try this pose on a flat surface and get good results. Besides bladder, all the organs of the body are getting good results through this pose.

Organs

> Bladder

Benefits

This pose is helpful in many ways:

Bridge pose increases the energy of the bladder

You will feel good and your bladder will become healthy through this pose

The muscles of the body and bladder will be relaxed and become healthy

Beginner tips

You need a flat surface for this pose. You must lay on the surface and bend your body from mid-section. Keep the head on the ground and the feet on the ground. Mid-section of the body must be raised to such a level that the legs are bent to 90 degrees. Keep your arms straight and remain in this pose for up to one minute.

Steps

1. Lay on the ground
2. Bend your legs and fold them from knees
3. Touch the ground with your feet and head
4. Your face must be facing the ceiling
5. Give the bend to the knees to almost 90 degrees
6. Let the body come down till head from the mid-section
7. Keep the arms straight
8. Your hands must be holding each other while in this pose
9. Continue till one minute before taking rest

Therapeutic applications

This pose increases health of bladder

Circulation of blood is improved to bladder which improves the function

Tension is released from bladder and muscles are relaxed

Precautions

You must not remain in this pose if you are feeling stress in muscles. Make sure that you perform this pose carefully so that stress from muscles could be avoided. When you feel tired or stressed then take rest and start this pose carefully and slowly. You must lay on ground or a flat surface for this pose. Avoid using soft places or your bed for the pose.

Poses For Ovaries, Prostate, Uterus

Yoga pose for Prostate: Butterfly Pose

This is a pose that is somehow easy compared to other poses as it targets the legs. It helps to relax and stretch the leg muscles after a long day of work.

Organs:

> Legs
> Muscles
> Feet
> Hand
> Knee

Benefits

> Helps in relaxing and stretching thighs after a long day of work e.g. runners, cyclers etc.
> Leads to the opening of hips and thigh which leads to flexibility.
> It stimulates digestive organs and reproduction
> Helps in reducing tiredness and stress

Beginner's tips

Proper padding around ankles is needed. The yoga will prevent your thighs to hurt and help you perform the exercise better. Also, you can roll up towels and put them under your thigh.

Steps

1. Begin by sitting in a position of a lotus pose also known as Padma Asana
2. Put your legs in a position that soles of the feet touch each other. You should bend your knees.

3. Put your legs in a position that is close to your pubic area as possible.
4. Hold your feet with your hand and sit with your back straight.
5. Breathe in and ensure that you place your hands on your knees.
6. Start breathing out as you press your thighs so that your knees touch the ground. Not everyone can do this, but one should not over exert himself and push down comfortably as far as you can
7. Breathe in and freely to make the knees come up
8. Breath out and re-do the same process 15-20 times
9. Speed up the low and rise up the thighs to help you relax the muscles. This is what leads to the name butterfly pose.

Therapeutic Application

It is a good posture for women especially during menstruation because it relieves discomfort and pain that is associated with the same.

It is of high benefit to women that have reached menopause

Exercising this pose regularly will benefit the kidney, prostate gland, and ovaries.

Precautions

Doctor's consultation is important before starting the exercise

It is important for the new beginners to do the exercise with the guidance of a trained instructor.

Yoga Pose for Uterus: Garland Pose

Garland pose is a kind of a pose that is meant for improving the digestive system. It mostly benefits thighs and also leads to the strengthening of the muscles.

Organs

> ➢ Thighs
> ➢ Hands
> ➢ Knees

Benefits

> ➢ Helps in the strengthening of the legs, ankles, knees, thighs and also spine.
> ➢ It results to effective digestion system and helps the body to release digestive matters well.

Beginner's tips

Use a chair. Sit on the chair, your legs perpendicular to your torso. Place the heels on the floor slightly further from the knees. Position your torso between your knees and lean ahead.

Steps

1. Face forward on the ground and squat keeping your feet on the ground. If you can't, keep your heels flat and use a folded blanket to support it.
2. Slowly separate your thighs wide enough so that you can lean on to your torso, and ensure that everything fits in. Put your hands together as you gently press your elbows against inner knees. This will make your front torso lengthen further as it presses.
3. Ensure you press your inner thighs against your torso. Put your arms on your legs and press your shins into your armpits. As you do this, try clasping your ankles as it will help the torso to lengthen further.
4. Stay in this position for like 30seconds and then slowly increase the time duration. Breathe out as you gently wake up.

Therapeutic Application

The exercise if recommended to pregnant women.

The pose helps to loosen the hip joint and also lead to labour. It is also good as it helps in relieving constipation.

Garland pose is recommended for pregnant women since it helps their body to prepare for labour.

Precautions

Individuals suffering from any form of lower back or knee injury should not pose.

Cow pose

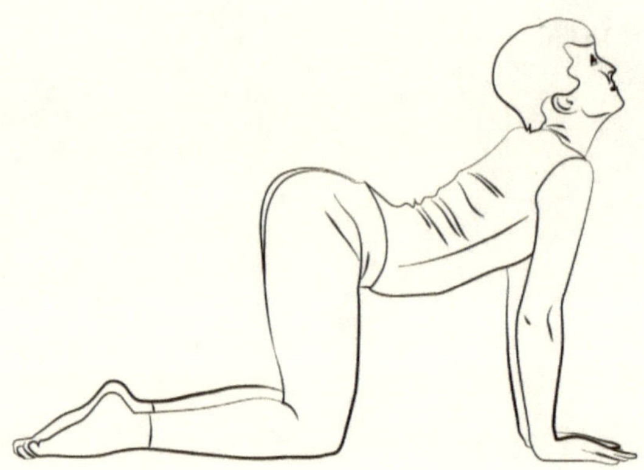

This pose actually acts as the counter pose type to a cat pose. It also provides a way to exercise of the spine.

Organs:

> Lower spine
> Hips
> Back as well as core muscles

Benefits:

> Enhance easier breathing by opening the lungs as well as the chest.
> It promotes a healthy spine due to the improvement of the posture.
> It facilitates the stretching of the hips, abdomen and the back region.

Beginner's tips:

Ensure that you adopt the right posture before you start the activity. Start with the easiest technique slowly before you introduce those that are complex. By doing this, you will prepare your body and muscles for the next level.

Steps:

1. Start kneeling on both your knees and hands; ensure that the position you are in is about three feet and well gazed in front of you. Ensure that all your knees are in a proper line with both of your wrists and hips and the shoulders as well as elbows are on the floor and perpendicular to each other.

2. Inhale as you lift your chest and tailbone in the position of the ceiling as you curve your back in a downward position on the floor. Start raising your head but don't force it into a back position of yours. At that position, fix your gaze in any spot you pick. Ensure that your knees are now down and maintain the perpendicular position of both your hands and legs on the floor.

3. Now start exhaling in a slow manner as you return to your normal position which was the original spot where you started. Ensure that you repeat the procedure several times to enhance flexibility.

Therapeutic Applications:

If the pose is properly conducted it stimulates various organs such as the gastrointestinal tract. This will lower the back pains and also reduce stress encountered by human beings. It is advisable to conduct such pose on daily life.

Precautions:

When you encounter any pain during the pose make sure you modify it by using the appropriate procedure like the one given above.

If you have encountered injury on the knee extend the time period of performing the pose or even avoid performing it and resume when you are well.

Crescent moon pose

This kind of pose involves both the pelvis and the legs to appear in the position of the parallel feet as the body trunk maintains a C-shaped curve to the sideway part of the body. The counterbalance is experienced by the legs through committing the body weight in a given foot direction.

Organs:

- Hands
- Hips
- Shoulders
- chest

Benefits:

- It is an energizing pose
- It stretches all sides of the body
- It builds the strength of the body
- Provides flexibility in the spine
- It enhances better circulation

Beginners tips:

1. The initial stage of the pose may be difficult if you are a beginner. As a beginner, you have to look for good crescent pose in order to avoid balance which is lost during the process. Pose for too long is not advisable since it may lead to injury and falling.

Steps:

2. Turn to a mountain pose
3. Lift your arms towards your shoulder in a sideway manner

4. Ensure you twist your arms into a ceiling face.
5. Inhale as you lift your arms to be above your head.
6. Ensure that your fingers are interlaced together as you point them upward. Make sure that your shoulders are relaxed in a downward manner as your arms turn close to your ears.
7. Inhale as you try to press the soles of your feet on the floor as you extend it through your fingertips.
8. Exhale and try to bend from your waist as you make sure you lean to the right.
9. Now try to press your hips in a gentle manner towards the left side. Make sure that you also press through both of your feet.
10. Look straight ahead as you point your head upwards.
11. Ensure you maintain this pose for at least 15 to 30 seconds.
12. Inhale as you make upright your torso
13. Repeat the above steps using the other side. Bring the arms in a downward manner as you exhale to ensure that the pose is released.

Therapeutic Applications:

It enhances the achievement of the lateral flexion with a great freedom in both the lumbar and the cervical spinal curves since there is a limited resistance of both the ribcage and sternum.

Precaution:

There is lower back problems or shoulder problems. Therefore minimize your stetch to avoid pains.

The cats pose:

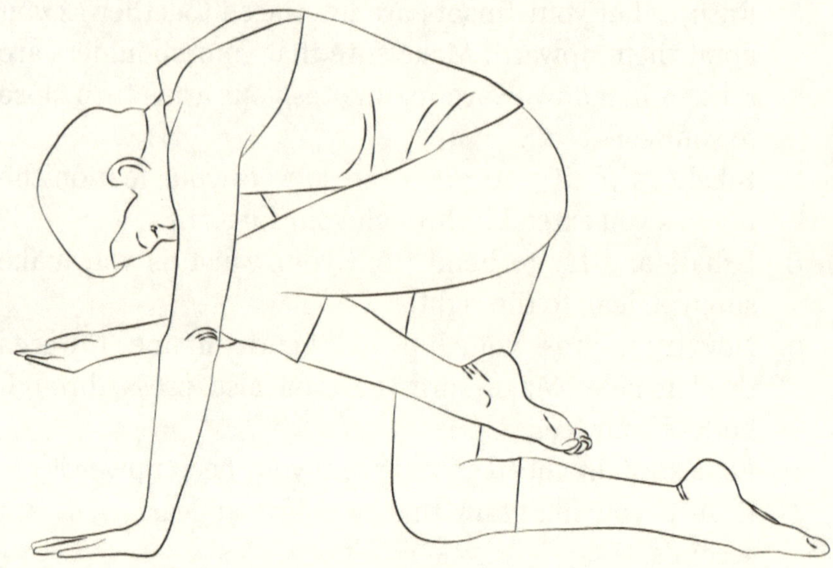

When you select yoga it is advisable that you enhance your enthusiasm for a little while. Ensure that you start with the beginner's style since this will assist you to prepare your body in order to perform those that are more complicated. By doing this, you will minimize the chance of suffering any tissue or ligament damage.

Organs:

> Hands
> Knees
> Shoulders
> Wrists
> Chest

Benefits

> It enhances the durability as well as the sturdiness of the spinal column.
> The individual posture is corrected while playing a significant role.

- ➢ The spine is reinvigorated together with the body internal organs.
- ➢ Assist in blood purification within the body.

Beginner's tips:

During the process you might experience difficulty around your top part of the upper back. You have to ask for help from your friend so that he or she places his hand above as well as between the blades of your shoulder. This will put you in a position of activating this part. Getting such help will enhance your interest and avoid disappointments.

Steps:

1. The first step is to get into a table top position using your hands while the knees are on the floor. Keep this kind of posture since it is very important to ensure that your knees are below your hips as well as wrists, shoulders and elbows. Ensure that all these parts are aligned with each other while remaining perpendicular to the floor. The head part must be in a centered position while your focus should be firmly locked on the floor.
2. The second step is to enhance exhaling while you round your spine in the position of the ceiling. Make sure that both your hands and knees remain intact to their positions and no movement should occur.
3. Ensure that now your head is released towards the part of the floor but make sure that you don't force your chin near the chest.
4. Lastly, inhale as you return your body in the form of the table top position which you started with originally. Repeat the same steps as many times as you wish to do so.

Therapeutic Application:

The pose enhances the release of stress in terms of therapeutic applications among other regular workouts.

It acts as the most widely stress relief method in most people in the world. More so, it is recommendable to practice the pose in order to reduce the amount of stress encountered.

Precaution:

In any event, you feel like having the head injury ensure that the head is in the direct line with the torso part and well maintained.

It is helpful if you have the yoga professional to give you proper guidance as you enhance the movements in order to perform the pose in the manner required.

Poses For Shoulder and Neck

Cow face arms for shoulders and neck

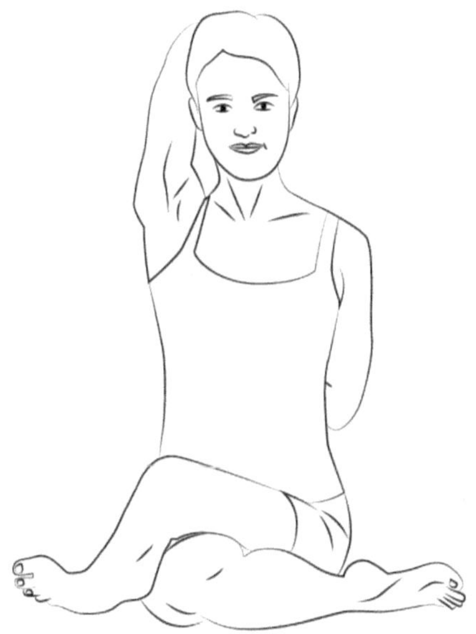

This pose is helpful for release of tension in muscles of neck and shoulders. You can perform it at any time as it is simple and effective. You can eliminate and reduce the pain in muscles of neck and shoulders by using this pose. Make sure that you are kneeling while in this pose for performing it easily and without problems.

Organs

- ➢ Neck
- ➢ Shoulders

Benefits

This pose eliminates tension from muscles of neck and shoulders

Flexibility of muscles in neck and shoulders is increased

Pain in muscles of neck is eliminated

You can reduce pain from shoulders through this pose

This pose is simple and easy for neck and shoulders

You can try this pose at any time for getting benefits

Beginner tips

You must tilt your body backwards in order to make the hands meet while in this pose. You must not put pressure or push the hands while in this pose. Make sure that you are not increasing stress on muscles while in this pose.

Steps

1. There are some steps which must be followed for this pose:
2. You must kneel on a hard surface like the floor
3. You must take the right arm and extend it towards the ceiling
4. Bend the right arm from elbow and take the right hand on the back side among shoulders
5. Take the left arm and bend it from elbow while using the down path
6. Try to hold the right and left hand at the back side of the body
7. When the hands meet then stay in this position for up to one minute
8. Continue to inhale and exhale while in this pose

Therapeutic applications

Tension from muscles in neck and shoulders is eliminated through this pose. You can use this pose for elimination of pain from neck and shoulders. You can apply this pose at any time when needed. You can stay in this pose for relaxation of muscles in neck and shoulders without inserting pressure. Strength and flexibility of muscles in neck and shoulders is increased by using this pose.

Precautions

Make sure that you are not trying hard and exerting pressure on your arms to make the hands meet at the back side. Try to tilt the body so that the hands could meet. If you feel pressure in the arms then return to normal position. This pose is good for elimination off tension from muscles and you must perform it with care for elimination of stress.

Point shoulder opener for neck and shoulders

This pose is helpful for increasing strength of shoulder and neck. You can relax the muscles of shoulder and neck by using this pose. You can start this pose at any time and stay in it for as long as you want for getting good results.

Organs

> Shoulders
> Neck

Benefits

This pose increases strength of muscles in neck

Strength of shoulders is increased through this pose

Muscles of neck will be relaxed

Relaxation of muscles in shoulders

This pose eliminates stress and tension from muscles in neck

Stress and tension from muscles in shoulders are eliminated

Beginner tips

You must find a straight place or an even floor for performance of this pose. You should use the ground and other tough places for this pose. Make sure to avoid extra pressure on your shoulders and neck while in this pose. Keep the muscles relaxed and flexible for getting benefits through the pose.

Steps

1. Lay on the ground on your back
2. Extend right arm outside at almost 90 degrees
3. Make sure that your palm is facing upwards
4. Take the left arm and hold the right hand and stay in this position
5. You must bend on left side while performing this pose
6. Stay in the pose. Inhale and exhale for some time

Therapeutic applications

This pose will eliminate tension from muscles from neck and shoulders

Flexibility of muscles in neck and shoulders will be increased

You will feel relaxed and comfortable as a result of this pose

Precautions

You must complete all the steps in this pose to make sure that there is no stress. Avoid fast speed as this will cause stress on the muscles. Make sure that you are working in this pose with relaxation and care. Stay in this pose for as long as you feel good and then return to normal position before starting another set.

Shoulder opener on blocks for neck and shoulders

This pose uses blocks on which the arms will rest. It is good for increasing strength of muscles of neck and shoulders. You can perform this pose at any time for relaxation of muscles of neck and shoulders. This pose is also helpful for elimination of pain from muscles of neck and shoulders.

Organs

- ➢ Neck
- ➢ Shoulders
- ➢ Benefits

Benefits:

This pose stretches the muscles of neck and shoulders

It increases flexibility of muscles of neck and shoulders

Stress and tension from muscles of neck are eliminated by this pose

Tension from muscles in shoulders is reduced by using this pose

Beginner tips

You must perform this pose slowly and make sure that the body is not under stress. Use simple clothes in which you can bend easily. You can use some cloth on the floor for performance of this pose. Flat surface is good for performance of this pose.

Steps

1. In order to perform this pose you must follow these steps:
2. Kneel on your knees
3. Place two blocks in front and make sure they are not moving
4. Place your elbows on the blocks and keep them in this place
5. Join your hands together as in prayer and bend the arms from elbows
6. Place the head between the arms and in the downward direction

7. Your hands must be on the back side and your head must be in the front side
8. Stay in this pose for up to one minute before returning to normal position

Therapeutic applications

This pose is helpful for elimination of stress from muscles of neck and shoulders. Pain from shoulders and neck is eliminated or reduced by using this pose. You can perform this pose at any time for increasing strength of muscles in neck and shoulders.

Precautions

Make sure that you perform all the steps in this pose with care. Reduce tension while in this pose and stay for as long as you feel easy. Continue to inhale and exhale while in this pose.

Poses For Sacrum

Legs Up the wall pose

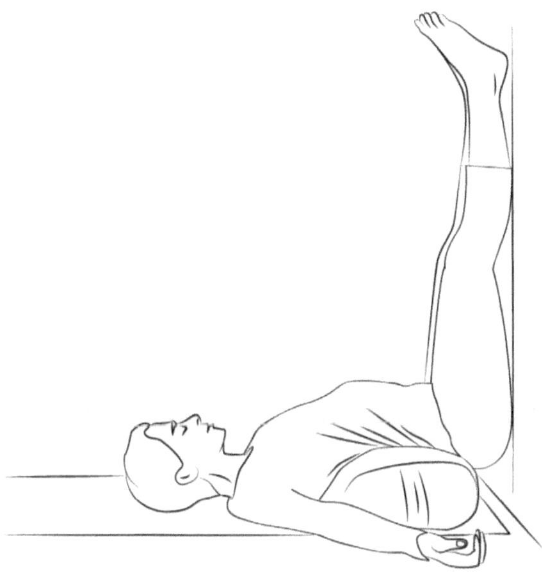

The 'legs up the wall' posture is one of the most nourishing and calming poses and people will find it very essential once they start doing it. This pose reduces anxiety and helps to calm our mind and body. The Sanskrit word is 'Viparita Karani'.

Benefits:

It helps to regulate blood flow.

Digestion process is improved

Reduces stress

It is a relief for a mild back pain.

A migraine and headache relief are provided

Keeps us young and vital

Eyes and ear problems will be taken care of.

Reduces testicular, semen and ovarian problems in men and women respectively.

Swollen ankles will get a relief.

Beginner's tip:

While breathing, bring the heads of the thigh bones towards the wall which helps in releasing your belly and spine.

Steps:

1. This pose should be done facing the wall and you can get a thick mat or a firm bolster for the support.
2. Determine the height of the support and also its distance from the wall. If your body is stiff the support should be lower and kept farther away from the wall. Use a higher support if you are flexible.
3. Sit sideways so that your right side should be facing the wall. The right side would be preferable for right-handers. As you exhale, swing your legs up onto the wall and your shoulders and head should be resting on the mat. There is a chance of facing a slight difficulty in doing this but this becomes easy after carrying out few times.
4. The front portion of your torso should round up and tilt backwards to lie down. You will feel a stretch from your pubis to your shoulder.
5. Tilt your head downwards and at the same time avoid your chin touching your chest.
6. The shoulder blades should be opened to allow your arms to rest beside the body with palms facing upwards.
7. Release the weight of the torso to keep the legs firm and straight and hold this pose for at least 7 minutes.

Precaution:

Do not perform this pose while menstruating.

Return back to the sitting position if you experience any tingling in your feet.

Pigeon Pose

Pigeon pose can be helpful in finding a relief for the stress and back pain. It also reduces trauma, fear and anxiety. Pigeon pose is one of the best poses for the open hip. In Sanskrit, it is called 'Eka Pada Rajakapotasana'.

Benefits:

Calms your mind

Stretches the thighs, groins and hip flexors.

Balances your core

It also opens the hips.

Helps people with urinary disorder

Hips get more flexible.

Reduces lower back ache and stiffness

Internal organs get stimulated

The most important benefit is that it opens the hip and releases all sort of negative energy from your body.

Beginner's tips:

You can rest on your elbows or hands by staying up higher.

Many people will find it difficult to rest on their foreheads, so you can make a cushion of your hand.

Steps:

1. Start on all fours and bring your right knee and place it behind your right hand. The ankle should be placed somewhere in front of the left hip.

2. Slide your left leg back and point the toes by straightening your knee.
3. To keep your hips square, draw your legs in towards each other.
4. Lower yourself down and if needed use your right buttock to keep your hips levelled.
5. On inhaling, lift your upper body and concentrate on your fingertips, hands shoulder width apart and open your chest.
6. Exhale, Lower your upper body to the floor and rest your forehead on the ground.
7. Remain in this position for a couple of breaths and on exhaling, try to release your tension in your right hip.
8. Balance your weight on both your legs and then change the sides.

Precaution:

Be careful of your knees, if your knees hurt, bring it closer to the left hip or underneath your right buttock.

Try to bring your left hip completely to the floor and keep your hips levelled. This will avoid further problems with your hip.

Monkey Pose

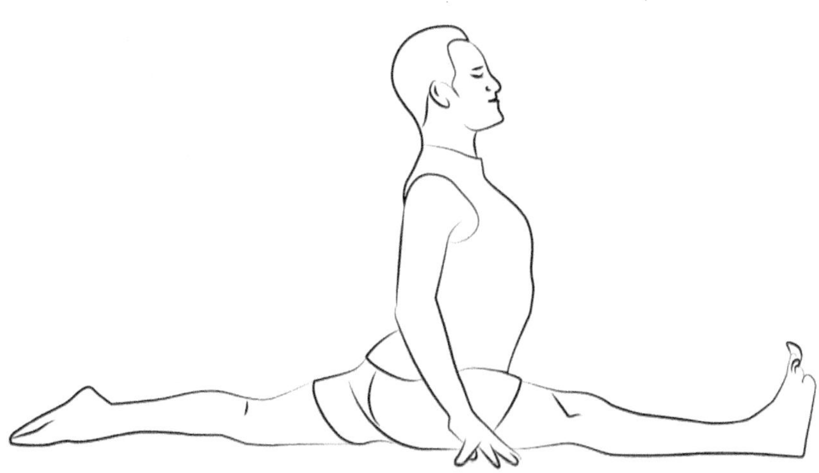

Monkey pose is also known as the 'split' and is named by the yoga practitioners. This monkey pose resembles the advanced leg stretch and helps in making your hips more flexible. The monkey pose got its name from the Hindu monkey god 'Hanuman'. In Sanskrit, it is known as 'Hanumanasana'.

Benefits:

Monkey pose keeps your legs supple and flexible and reduces the risks of injuries.

Stimulates the organs in the abdominal region and improves the overall functioning.

Abdominal muscles will also get toned in this exercise.

It opens up the hips on practicing it every day increases the overall flexibility and alignment.

It also stretches both thighs and hamstrings.

Beginner's tips:

Lift the shoulder blades firmly after pressing the back foot on the floor to increase the length of the spine and torso.

Steps:

1. Put your knees on the floor and step your right foot in front of your left knee and rotate your right thigh.
2. On exhaling, leave your torso forward and concentrate on the palms fixed on the floor. Slide your left knee back and descend the right thigh towards the floor at the same time.
3. Push your right toe away from your torso and gradually turn the leg inward as it straightens to bring the knee cap towards the ceiling.
4. Start pressing the left knee back and descend the front of the left thigh.
5. Centre of the right knee should point directly towards the ceiling.
6. Lift the foot towards the ceiling and thus, make the front leg active.
7. Stretch the arms up towards the ceiling and remain in this position for about a minute.
8. Then press your hands to the floor and turn the front leg out which returns the front heel and back knee to the initial point.
9. Repeat this after reversing your legs.

Precaution:

Practice this pose carefully as you may hurt your hamstring or cause groin injuries.

The cat pose

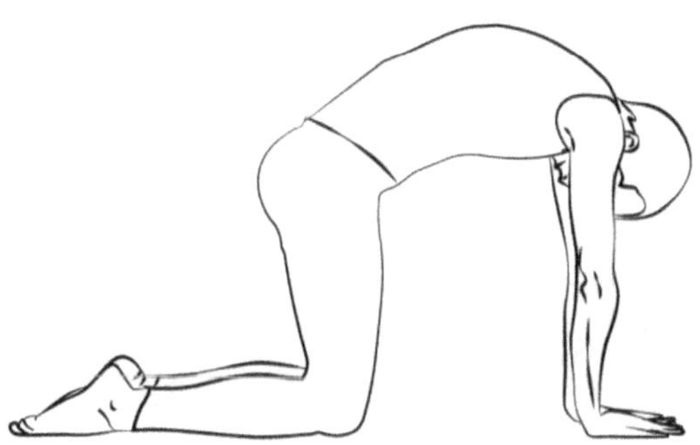

Can you ever imagine that even the pet cats can teach us various lessons in reducing back pain! Cat pose or otherwise called as Marjari asana in Sanskrit is an excellent pose which helps in reducing back pain.

Benefits:

Improves the digestion process

Abdomen muscles get toned

Flexibility is experienced in spine

Reduces back pain

Blood circulation is improved

Beginner's Tip:

If you have any problems in bringing your body in this pose, you can ask a friend to lay a hand just above and between the shoulder blades to help you activate this area.

Steps:

1. Make your body in the form of a table and rest both hands and legs on the floor. This should be in a position in which your back forms the table top and your hands and feet from the legs of the table.
2. The hands rested on the floor must be perpendicular to it and they should be directly under the shoulders and flat on the ground. The knees should be hip-width apart.
3. Look straight and as you inhale, your chin should be raised and tilt your head back. Then raise your tailbone and push your navel downwards. You will feel a slight tingle on your buttocks.
4. Take long deep breaths in this pose and as you exhale, drop your chin to your chest slowly and arch your back up as much as you can.
5. Relax your buttocks and hold this pose for some time.
6. Then return to your previous table-like position and relax.
7. Try doing this five or six times to experience the changes and the most important tip you should keep in your mind is to carry out this movement slowly and gracefully.

Precaution:

Before practicing marjari asana, it would be best to consult a doctor if you are suffering from any abdomen, back or neck problems.

The Cow Pose

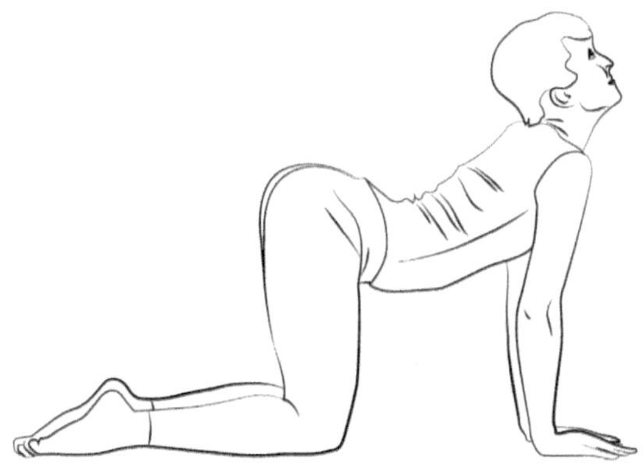

They are usually performed at the beginning of the class and is paired with cat pose to form vinyasa. The term vinyasa is defined as 'breathe synchronized movement'. But cow pose alone in Sanskrit is called 'Bitilasana'. Cow in Sanskrit is called 'Bitila' and the pose means 'asana'.

Benefits:

This pose is a very good stress reliever.

It massages the internal organs and the spine.

Stretches the neck and front of the torso.

It calms the mind.

Reduces back pain.

It also improves balance and posture.

Beginner's tip:

To avoid injuries on your neck, it should be broadened across the shoulders and the shoulders must be drawn away from the ears. It would best if you could do this pose in front of the mirror for correct alignment.

Steps:

1. The first position is almost equal to that of the cat pose. Both the hands and knees should be in a table like position. Make sure your wrists, elbows, and shoulders are in line and perpendicular to the ground and your knees should be set directly below your hips.
2. Spread your fingers on the mat and check if the crease of your wrist is in line with the mat. The position of your head should also be taken care of and must be placed in a neutral position, your gaze resting on the floor.
3. Inhale, and lift your sitting bones towards the ceiling along with the chest, allowing your belly to sink towards the floor.Lift your head straight to look up.
4. Exhale, returning back to the previous table-like position.
5. Repeat this few times, about 10 -15 times, to experience the benefits.
6. This is often paired with the cat pose to form vinyasa.

Precautions:

Keep your head in line with the torso if you have a neck injury. Protect your neck by dropping the shoulders away from the ears.

The Bridge Pose

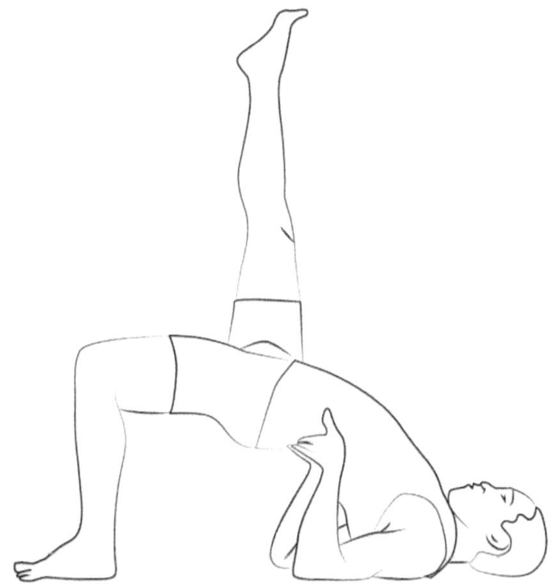

(Variation One legged Bridge Pose)

The Sanskrit name for this pose is 'Setu Bandha Sarvangasana'. Setu means 'Bridge', Bandha means 'Bind' and asana means 'posture'. This pose resembles a bridge and hence the name.

Benefits:

It is very good for asthma patients.

Helpful for high blood pressure, sinusitis, and osteoporosis.

It helps improve digestion.

Reduces anxiety and calms the brain.

Very essential for people experiencing back pain and also strengthens back muscles.

Reduces thyroid problems.

Stretches the upper part of the body including chest, neck and also the spine.

Beginner's tip:

Get the help of a partner to learn the correct action of the top thighs in a backbend. When lifting the top of the shoulders towards the ears, push the inner shoulder blades away.

Steps:

1. Lie on your back to begin with the exercise.
2. Fold your knees and set your feet on the floor. Keep this at a distance of 10-12 inches away from your pelvis with knees and ankles in a straight line.
3. Keep in mind that your arms should be kept beside the body with the palms facing down.
4. Slowly lift your lower back, middle back and upper back on inhaling and gently roll on the shoulders.
5. Make your chin touch your chest without bringing your chin down.
6. Support the weight with your arms, shoulders and feet. The thighs should be parallel to each other and to the floor.
7. If you think you could lift your back a little more with your fingers, you can use your palm.
8. Relax and keep breathing easily.
9. Try holding this posture for a minute or so, and release your body on exhaling.
10. Relax and then try this a few more times.

Precaution:

For safety first, this pose should be done only if you don't have any neck and back injuries. Practice it under the supervision of a teacher.

Peacock pose

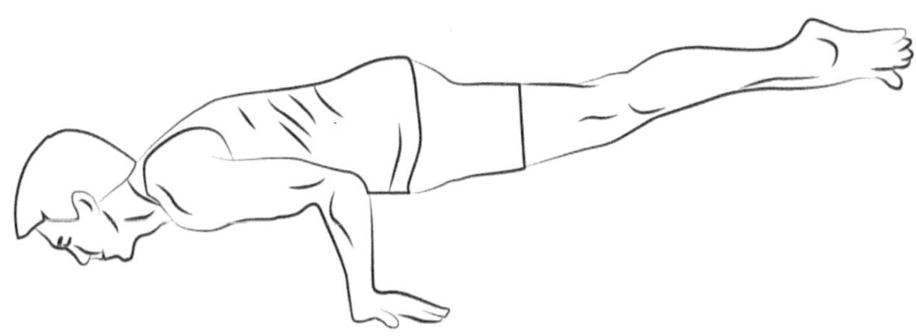

If you want to eat anything you want and have a perfect digestion, then the peacock pose is the best pose for you. In this pose, you exert pressure on the digestive organs. This is done by balancing the weight of your torsos on using your arms. This cuts off blood supply to the digestive organs for a moment.

When you release the pose, what flows into your digestive organs is fresh blood rich in oxygen. This improves their general functioning. With the compression experienced also, this helps in removing any that may be stuck.

Benefits:

Reduces stress

It is a relief for a mild back pain.

It helps in regulation of blood flow.

Digestion process is improved

A migraine and headache relief are provided

Keeps you young and energized.

Eyes and ear problems will be taken care of.

Reduces testicular, semen and ovarian problems in men and women respectively.

Clears any obstacles along the digestive organs' tract.

Beginner's tip:

Taking a deep breath, balance your weight on your hands while on a horizontal position. Make sure the rest of your body does not touch the ground.

Steps:

1. Once you have successfully balanced your torsos on your arms, hold the pose for some few seconds before releasing it and beginning all over again. Do not hold it for long until your body stiffens.
2. Make sure that you use a smooth surface to place your hands once you don't want to hurt your palms with rough floors. Ensure also that you are able to breathe freely. There is a chance of facing a slight difficulty in doing this at first if you have a large body but this becomes easy after carrying out few times.
3. Tilt your head downwards and at the same time avoid your chin touching the floor.
4. Release the weight of the torso to keep the legs firm and straight and hold this pose for at least 7 minutes.

Precaution:

If you experience any discomfort, please release the weight on your hands by lying on your tummy to release the stress.

Do not perform this pose while pregnant.

Peacock pose can be helpful in finding a relief for the stress and back pain. It also reduces trauma, fear and anxiety. Peacock pose is one of the best poses for the perfect digestion.

Wind Relieving Pose

This is another perfect pose those struggling with sluggish digestion, or those that experience trapped wind. Also known as the purvana – mukta – asana, this pose helps release gastrointestinal gas, relieving stomach upsets and constipation. The The Sanskrit word pavana means air or wind andmukta means freedom or release, therefore this is the "wind relieving posture"

Benefits:

Improves digestion

Relieves your mind of stress

Stretches the back, groins and hip flexors.

Eliminates back pains.

Lengthens the spine.

Relieves the body against constipation

Reduces lower back ache and stiffness

Internal organs get stimulated

The most important benefit is that it increases digestion and enables fresh flow of blood to the organs.

Beginner's tips:

You can use the Vinyasa pose to build a sequence that leads to this pose.

Difficulty is rather easy, as it only involves lying on your back as a preliminary procedure.

Steps:

1. Lying on your back, inhale both knees into your chest. Wrap the arms around the knees, holding on to opposite elbows, forearms, wrists or fingers.
2. Tuck the chin into the chest with the head on the floor. Press the sacrum and tailbone down into the floor as you pull the knees into the chest using the arms.
3. Press the shoulders and the back of the neck down into the floor, trying to get the back and whole spine flat to the floor. Relax the legs, feet and hips.
4. Breathe and hold for 4-8 breaths, breathing deeply into the belly, actively pressing it against the thighs on the inhalation.
5. Hold the inhaled breath for a few seconds then exhale while bringing the right leg to the floor.
6. Lie flat on the back in the shava-asana for a few seconds then repeat beginning with the left leg
7. To release: exhale and release the arms and legs to the floor.

Precaution:

Avoid this pose in case you just had abdominal surgery as it could cause further complications.

If you have hernia, it could worsen the situation.

Corpse pose

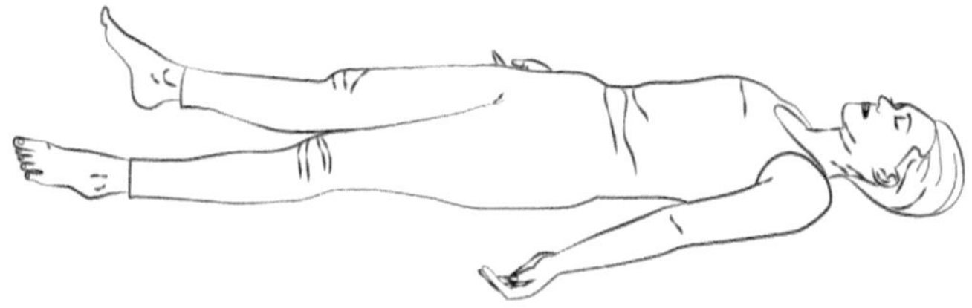

After working out in a yoga class, the corpse pose offers the best energy restoration. Also known as Final relaxation pose and Savasana in Sankrit, this pose can be very tough to learn despite looking easy in the first place. "Savasana" (shah-VAHS-uh-nuh), comes from two words. The first is "Sava" (meaning "corpse"), and the second is "asana" (meaning "pose"). Savasana implies a depth of release that goes beyond simple relaxation. This resting pose takes your yoga practice to a place where you can completely let go.

Benefits:

Lowers blood pressure.

Decelerates the rate of heart beat.

Slows down the rate of respiration.

Decreases the rate of metabolism in the body.

Decreases the rate of muscle tension.

Reduces occurrence of headaches

Provides relief from insomnia and tiredness.

Increases self- confidence.

Improves concentration and memory.

Raises your energy levels.

Provides relief against anxiety and and panic.

Reduces nervous tension in the body.

Increases body productivity.

Beginner's tips:

Lie on your back with your arms along your sides and your legs straight. Ensure you rest your body on a soft surface, and a good recommendation would be a blanket.

Steps:

1. Let your breath continue naturally.
2. Allow your body to feel heavy on the ground.
3. Working from the soles of your feet up to the crown of your head, consciously release every body part, organ, and cell.
4. Relax your face. Let your eyes drop deep into their sockets. Invite peace and silence into your mind, body, and soul.
5. Stay in Savasana for five minutes for every 30 minutes of your practice.
6. To exit the pose, deepen your breath first, then bring gentle movements and awareness back to your body, nibbling your fingers and your toes in the process. You can roll to your side and rest in that position for some few seconds. Taking a deep breath, raise yourself gently to a sitting position.

Precaution:

If you have discomforts like on your back, you may have to practice the supported version of the corpse pose.

For pregnant women, they should ensure that their head and chest are raised in the pose by using a cushion.

Work within your limits, and if you have any medical concerns, contact your doctor before beginning practicing this pose.

Standing forward fold pose

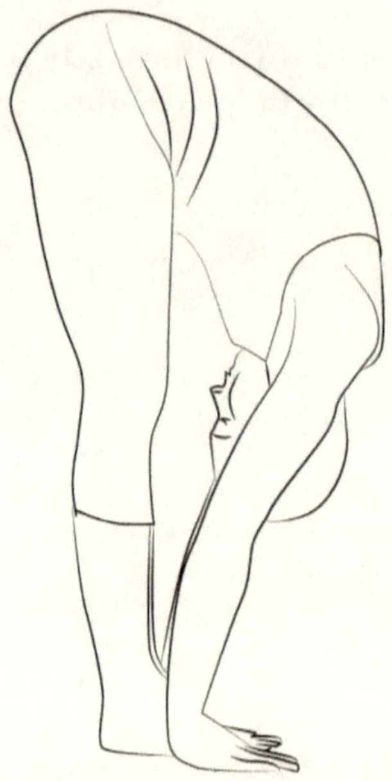

The standing forward pose, also known as Uttanasana (ooh-tuhn-AHS-uh-nuh) is a pose that combines both the benefits of inversions and those of forward folds. The literal translation of its Sanskrit name is "intense stretch pose." This comes from three Sanskrit words:

"Ut" — meaning "intense"

"Tan" — meaning "to stretch"

"Asana" — meaning "pose"You drop your head below you heart, bringing a calming effect in the process.This type of pose works to relieve stress, as it deeply stretches your hamstring and calves.

Benefits:

Provides relief against headaches.

Relieves stress.

It is a relief for insomnia and fatigue.

It helps in regulation of blood flow.

Calms the brain

A migraine and headache relief are provided

Keeps you young and energized.

Provides solutions to mild depressions.

Beginner's tip:

From Tadasana, take a deep breath while bending your hips to lengthen the front of your torso.

Steps:

1. Clasp your elbows with your arms bent. Let the crown of your head hang down, then press your heels into the floor and lift your sit bones toward the ceiling. Turn the tops of your thighs slightly inwards. Be sure not to lock your knees.
2. Lift and lengthen with each inhalation. Release deeper into the pose with each exhalation. Hold for up to a maximum of one minute, or as long as you are able to without compromising comfort.
3. To release this pose, draw down through your tailbone while inhaling then smoothly rise up to a standing position.
4. Return to Tadasana again and repeat this for 5 – 10 times in a single session.

Precaution:

The standing forward fold pose requires patience and a lot of practice in order to be able to exercise it correctly. It can take months or even years to successfully reach the deepest variations this pose has to offer.

Injuring yourself can occur easily if you push your body too much to attain this pose too early in the program.

If you are not flexible enough to exercise this pose in proper alignment, use a block to support your hands. You can also bend your knees at the beginning until you are able to do it with legs straight.

Those with back pains or injuries are specifically recommended to practice this pose while knees are bent to avoid further complications.

Reclining big toe pose

Are you a person who likes cycling, swimming, playing sports and lifting weights? Then you are quite familiar with tight hamstrings. These muscles are prone to stiffening when underused, and yet ironically, they also stiffen when overused.

Practicing the reclining big toe pose on a regular basis helps to increase the flexibility of these muscles, reducing the risk of getting pulled hamstrings. This pose, also known as Supine big toe pose and named in Sanskrit as "Supta Padangusthasana" (SOOP-tah pahd-ahng-goosh-TAHS-uh-nuh), comes from four words:

"Supta" — meaning "reclining"

"Pada" — meaning "foot"

"Angusta" — meaning "big toe"

"Asana" — meaning "pose"

Benefits:

Helps in opening the hips.

Reduces lower back pains.

Stimulates the prostate gland.

Improves digestion.

Can be used as a therapeutic for sciatica, high blood pressure and flat feet.

It stretches the calves and the groin.

 Strengthens the knees.

Can be therapeutic for infertility.

Beginner's tips:

To exercise this pose, you need a yoga strap, but if you can't get your hands on that, even a towel or a belt can be useful. Just an important point to note when using these other alternatives is that you need to avoid flexible or stretchy straps. The band should be held taut for the best effect.

Steps:

1. Lie on your back with your legs extended and arms resting at your sides. Relax your breath and let your thoughts settle down.
2. With an exhalation, bend your right knee and hug your thigh to your chest. Keep your left leg extended along the floor. Wrap the strap around the ball of your right foot and grasp one end of the strap in each hand. Keep your grip soft, but not loose.
3. Exhaling, reach through your heel to straighten your knee, extending your heel to the ceiling. Keep your right foot flexed and your buttocks equally balanced on the floor. Lift through the ball of your right big toe.
4. Draw slightly down on the strap. As you do, let the head of your thigh bone (the part of the bone that connects in the hip socket) release and rest in your pelvis. Feel your lower back press into the ground.
5. Press your shoulder blades lightly into the floor and broaden across your collarbones. Lengthen the back of your neck. Relax the muscles of your buttocks on the floor.

6. Softly gaze at your right big toe or at a single spot on the ceiling if you can't see your toe.
7. Hold this position for 1-3 minutes.
8. Exhale as you draw your knee into your chest and let go of the strap. Then, release your leg completely and extend it along the floor.
9. Repeat on the opposite side for the same length of time.

Precaution:

If you are experiencing diarrhea or headaches, do not practice this pose.

For people with high blood pressure, ensure that you first rest your heads and neck on a soft and firm blanket.

Pyramid pose

This is standing yoga that comes with three movements: the forward bending, backward bending, as well as balancing. Combining all these three movements requires deep focus and a very clear mind if you are to make the most out of it.

Its Sanskrit name, "Parsvottanasana" (PARZH-voh-tahn-AHS-uh-nuh), comes from four words:

"Parsva" — meaning "side" or "flank"

"Ut" — meaning "intense"

"Tan" — meaning "to stretch"

"Asana" — meaning "pose"

Benefits:

It's helpful in stretching the shoulders and hamstring.

Builds a balance and complete body co-ordination.

Calms the mind.

Stretches the spine.

Improves postural habits.

Stretches the chest and hips.

It is therapeutic for flat feet.

It stimulates abdominal organs hence improves digestion.

Reduces the chances of pulling your hamstring.

Beginner's tips:

Begin standing at the top of your mat or blanket with your arms at your sides in Tadasana. Slowly turn to the left and open your feet to about 3 to 4 feet apart. While placing your hands on your hips, Turn your right foot 90 degrees so the toes point to the top of the mat/blanket. Point your left toes at the top-left corner of your mat, turned about 60 degrees.

Steps:

1. Keeping your feet in place, gradually turn your entire torso to face the same direction as your front foot.
2. While squaring your hips at the top of the mat, draw your left hip slightly forward.
3. Inhale as you reach your arms out to the sides. As you breathe out, reach your arms behind your back. Clasp each elbow with the opposite hand
4. On an inhalation, ensure you elongate your torso. When exhaling, fold at the hips and extend your torso over your front leg. Keep the crown of your head extending forward and your tailbone reaching behind you. Be sure to fold from the hip, not the waist.
5. Ground down through the heel of your back foot. Try to stare at your big toe.
6. Hold for up to one minute.
7. Press firmly through your back heel and slowly lift your torso to release this pose. You can then change the position of your feet, and repeat on the opposite side.

Precaution:

If you have hamstring injury, refrain from this pose as it may worsen the situation and derail your recovery.

Persons with injured shoulders or wrists are advised not to practice the full version of this pose.

Pregnant women and those with back injuries or high blood pressure are advised to practice the pyramid pose with their hands resting against the wall.

Remember to work at your pace and avoid straining your body with the full version if you are not able to.

Poses for Groins

Garland Pose

The garland pose is a squatting pose which will develop the digestive system.

Organs

- ➤ Groins
- ➤ Legs
- ➤ Ankles
- ➤ Knees

Benefits

The garland pose can support the body in several different ways such as being beneficial to the legs as well as the tummy.

Extends the ankles, groins as well as the back torso.

It helps the groin and enhances the digestive system, assisting the entire body to expel waste matter effectively.

Beginner's Tips

A beginner's tip for garland pose contains utilizing a prop similar to a folded cover or bolster for support. You can even use a chair rather than dong the asana on the ground. Take a seat on the chair with the legs perpendicular to the torso. Heels must be put on the ground, somewhat in front of the knees.

Steps

1. Squat with the feet as close jointly as can be Split the thighs a bit wider than the torso.
2. Exhaling, trim the torso ahead and also fit it comfortably between the thighs.
3. Push your elbows against your own inner knees, taking the palms along Resist the knees into the elbows.
4. Once again, push the inner thighs against the edges of the torso.

5. Access your hands ahead, now swing them to the sides
   and also notch the shins into the armpits.
6. Push your fingertips to the ground, or even reach
   around the outside of your ankles and also clasp the
   back heels.
7. Maintain the positioning for at least 30 seconds to one
   minute, then breathe in, straighten the knees, then
   stand.

Therapeutic Applications

This pose is usually advised to pregnant women.

This pose can be a suggested pose for pregnant women
because it helps their body prepare for work.

The pose is recognized to release the hip joint also is proven to
bring on labor.

The pose is usually a great pose to ease constipation.

Precautions

Never perform this pose if there are a recent or even long-
term lower back or knee injuries.

Usually, work within your variety of limitations and
capabilities.

Having any kind of medical issues, meet with a doctor before
practicing yoga.

Low Lunge Pose

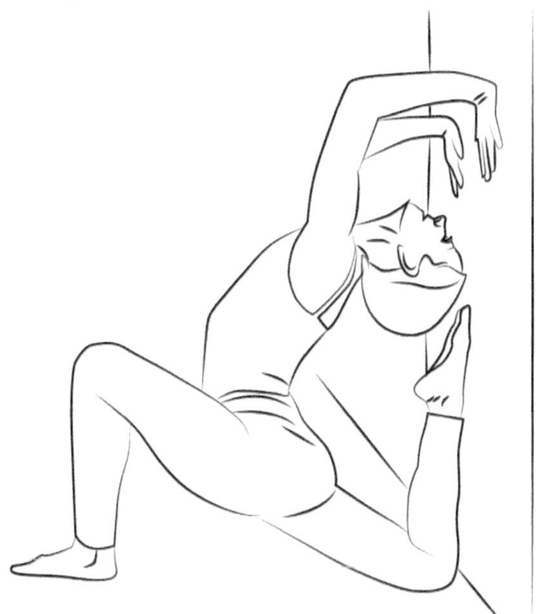

The Low Lunge is a great yoga pose. It helps to boost the strength as well as flexibility in your hips, legs, back, arms, abs, shoulder and knees.

Organs

- ➢ Groins
- ➢ Knees
- ➢ Arms
- ➢ Back

Benefits

Releases stress in your hips.

Extends the hamstrings, quads, as well as groin.

Improves the knees.

Assists you to grow mental concentration.

Beginner's Tips

To boost balance, perform this pose in a wall. Push the large toe of the forward foot against the wall then expands the arms up, fingertips to the wall surface.

Steps

1. Begin in Downward Facing Dog Pose.
2. On an exhalation, move the right foot ahead and put it beside the right thumb.
3. Lower the left knee to the ground, being sure to put it on the hips.
4. Bring up the torso and sweep the arms above the head with the palms fronting each other, putting the biceps beside the ears.
5. Now enable the hips to calm forwards and also down unless you sense a stretch in the front of the left leg as well as psoas.
6. Bring the tailbone did towards the earth. Start to get the thumbs into the back side plane of the body.
7. Stay here, or bring up the back knee off the mat for the full Crescent Lunge.
8. Finally, set the arms down on the mat as well as move back to Downward Facing Dog Pose Do again with the left leg forwards.

Therapeutic Applications

It is recommended for those who suffer from sciatica because it extends the hamstrings and also leg muscle tissues.

This pose is good for the heart. It stretches as well as stimulates the lower body.

Precautions

Hypertension.

Knees injury.

People with shoulder issues should never raise their hands above their head, instead putting their arms on their front thigh.

Tree Pose

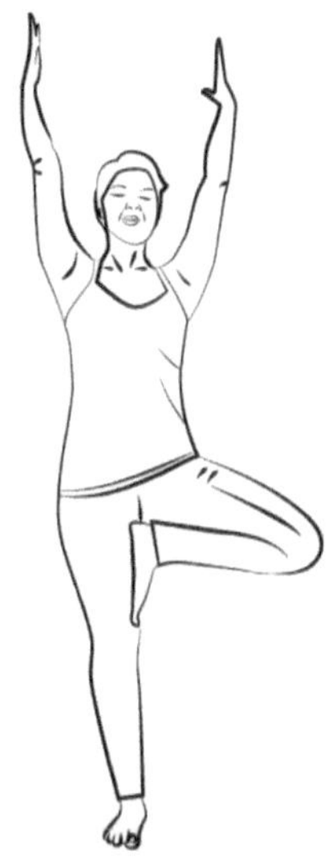

This pose helps to make the legs, ankles as well as feet stronger along with making hips and knees a lot more flexible.

Organs

> Groins
> Ankles
> Knees

Benefits

Boosts feeling of balance Reduces sciatica, as well as decreases flat feet, Stretches the whole body Makes the hips and knees a lot more flexible.

Beginner's Tips

If the raised foot has a tendency to slip down the inner standing thigh, place a folded tight mat between the raised-foot sole along with the standing internal thigh.

Steps

1. Start in mountain pose.

2. Move the weight on the left foot since the right leg is curved.
3. Relax the sole of the right feet beside the inside of left leg as much as possible but far from the knee.
4. The toes of the foot need to be pointed downwards Join the palms with each other at the upper body just like prayer pose.
5. Push the sole of the right foot against the inner of the left leg as well as maintain the curved right leg relaxed.
6. The sole of the left feet needs to be pushed into the ground Breathe while raising the hands over the head, with palms along and also stretched out by the fingers.
7. The crown of the head would be towards the roof and also gaze at the fixed position ahead of you.
8. Imagine you are going in upward, downward as well as outward at the same time.
9. Stay in this pose for fifteen to thirty seconds then return to mountain pose.
10. Do again steps from two to nine with the other leg.

Therapeutic Applications

It's highly recommended for those who want Stretches of shoulders and chest.

Great for improving thighs, calves, ankles, as well as the spine.

Precautions

Any kind of damage to the knees.

New injury of the hips.

Low blood pressure levels.

High blood pressure levels: Do not bring up hands over head.

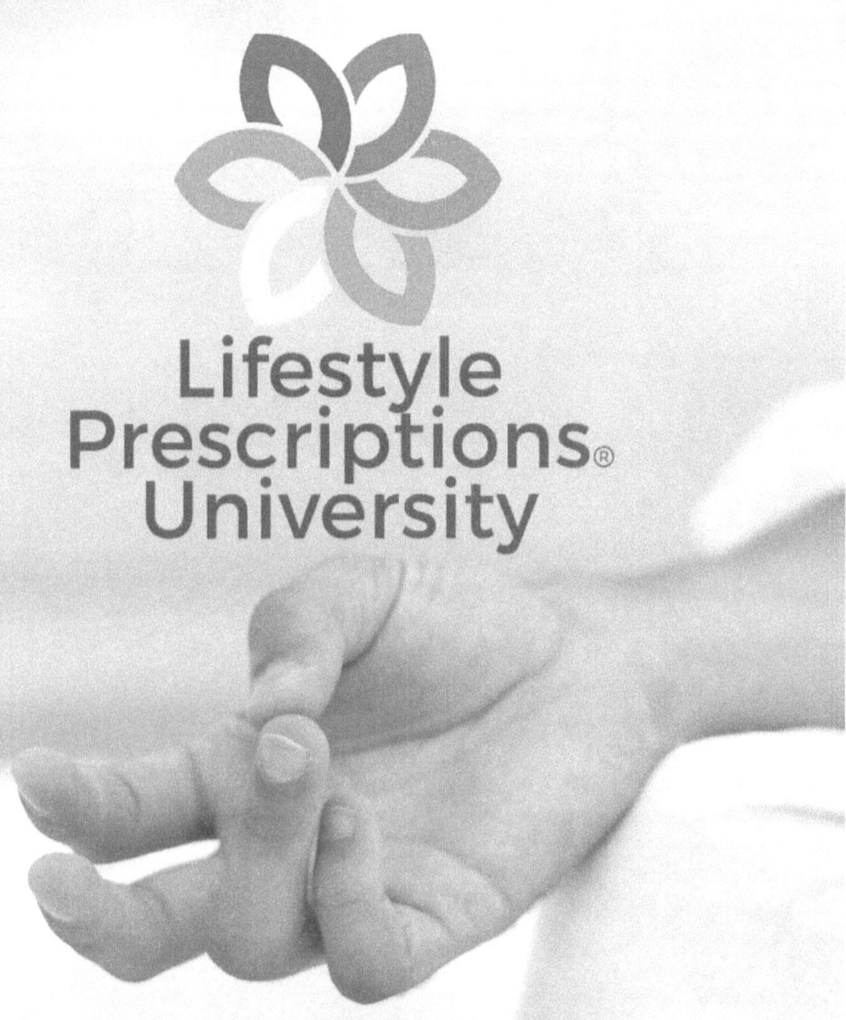

- Learn about certificate and degree programs at:
  https://lifestyleprescriptions.tv/phd

- Download the book "The 6 Root-Causes Of All Symptoms":
  https://lifestyleprescriptions.tv/book

- Watch the Lifestyle Prescriptions® 101 Video Course at:
  https://lifestyleprescriptions.tv/101

www.ingramcontent.com/pod-product-compliance
Lightning Source LLC
Chambersburg PA
CBHW062139150726
47991CB00006B/2104